TABLE OF CONTENTS

Quinoa and Roasted Vegetable Stuffed Bell Peppers

Grilled Portobello Mushroom Caps with Spinach and Feta

Vegetable and Lentil Curry

Baked Salmon with Pesto and Roasted Potatoes

Mediterranean Chickpea Salad

Grilled Chicken and Vegetable Wraps

Quinoa and Black Bean Burrito Bowls

Roasted Vegetable and Hummus Sandwich

Baked Cod with Tomato and Olive Sauce

Spinach and Feta Frittata

Grilled Chicken and Pineapple Skewers

Lentil and Sweet Potato Shepherd's Pie

Baked Salmon with Mango Salsa

Greek Quinoa Salad

Grilled Chicken and Vegetable Kebabs with Tzatziki Sauce

Baked Sweet Potato Fries with Garlic Aioli

Vegetable and Tofu Stir-Fry with Brown Rice Noodles

Grilled Salmon and Asparagus Salad with Lemon Vinaigrette

Quinoa and Black Bean Stuffed Bell Peppers

Baked Chicken with Roasted Brussels Sprouts and Sweet Potatoes

Vegetable and Lentil Soup with Pesto

Mediterranean Chickpea Salad with Grilled Shrimp

Quinoa and Roasted Vegetable Grain Bowls

Baked Cod with Tomato and Olive Tapenade

Spinach and Feta Stuffed Chicken Breasts

Grilled Veggie and Hummus Wraps

Sweet Potato and Black Bean Burrito Bowls

Lentil and Vegetable Curry with Coconut Milk

Baked Salmon with Mango Salsa and Quinoa

Greek Quinoa Salad with Grilled Chicken

Roasted Vegetable and Egg Breakfast Sandwiches

Vegetable and Tofu Stir-Fry with Brown Rice Noodles and Peanut Sauce

Grilled Salmon and Asparagus Salad with Lemon Vinaigrette and Quinoa

Quinoa and Black Bean Stuffed Bell Peppers with Avocado Salsa

Baked Chicken with Roasted Brussels Sprouts, Sweet Potatoes, and Balsamic Glaze

Vegetable and Lentil Soup with Pesto and Whole-Grain Crackers

Mediterranean Chickpea Salad with Grilled Shrimp and Feta

Quinoa and Roasted Vegetable Grain Bowls with Avocado

Baked Cod with Tomato and Olive Tapenade and Roasted Potatoes

Spinach and Feta Stuffed Chicken Breasts with Roasted Vegetables

Grilled Veggie and Hummus Wraps with Quinoa

Sweet Potato and Black Bean Burrito Bowls with Brown Rice

CONCLUSION

Title Page

Myasthenia Gravis

A Complete Guide to Understanding, Managing, and Driving Myasthenia Gravis into Remission with Delicious Anti-Inflammatory Recipes and Diet Plans

By: Kelvin Dino

Copyright

INTRODUCTION

Myasthenia gravis is not transmissible nor hereditary. It usually appears later in life as a result of the body's antibodies attacking healthy muscle receptors. This prevents the release of a substance that causes muscles to contract. When a woman with myasthenia gravis transmits her antibodies to the foetus, the foetus may develop a transient type of myasthenia gravis. It usually goes away in two to three months.

Approximately 20 persons per 100,000 worldwide suffer with myasthenia gravis. The true figure might be higher because some individuals with milder cases might not be aware they have the illness. The number of Americans with myasthenia gravis at any given time is estimated to be 60,000.

Myasthenia gravis impairs the nerve-muscle transmission system. Muscle weakness results, which gets worse with movement and the passage of time. Double vision or drooping eyelids are frequently the initial symptoms. It could be difficult for you to speak, swallow, stand, and lift objects. Myasthenia Gravis (MG) is a complex and often misunderstood autoimmune disorder that can profoundly impact one's quality of life. However, with the right knowledge and support, individuals living with MG can not only manage their symptoms but also thrive and lead fulfilling lives.

Myasthenia Gravis: A Complete Guide to Understanding, Managing, and Driving Myasthenia Gravis into Remission with Delicious Anti-Inflammatory Recipes and Diet Plans is a comprehensive resource that aims to empower you with a deep understanding of MG, equipping you with the tools and strategies necessary to navigate this challenging condition. This book will help you find strategies to feel better, eat healthily while managing the disease, and lower your chance of developing further issues and complications in the future.

CHAPTER ONE

*Understanding
Myasthenia Gravis*

What Is Myasthenia Gravis?

A persistent neuromuscular disease called myasthenia gravis is a chronic condition that results in voluntary muscle weakening. Muscles in the face, throat, and diaphragm, as well as muscles attached to a person's bones, are considered voluntary muscles. They are necessary for breathing, eating, and making facial movements. They contract to move the arms and legs. Being an autoimmune illness, myasthenia gravis results from the body's defence mechanism unintentionally attacking healthy cells or proteins necessary for regular operation. There are situations when a person requires a ventilator to breathe because their breathing muscles weaken. This is referred to as a myasthenic crisis, and it calls for emergency medical attention right now. An illness, stress, surgery, or a bad drug reaction can all cause a myasthenic crisis. A myasthenic crisis affects 15–

25% of individuals with myasthenia gravis at least once, and up to 50% of those individuals may not be able to pinpoint a trigger.

The disorder may develop suddenly. It's possible that myasthenia gravis symptoms are not immediately identifiable. The extent of the underlying muscle weakness varies widely between people. Myasthenia gravis results in weakening in the skeletal muscles. These are the muscles that facilitate movement by attaching to your bones. Typically, myasthenia gravis affects the muscles in your neck, arms, legs, and eyes. Men and women of diverse racial and ethnic backgrounds are affected by myasthenia gravis. It affects young adult women (under 40) and older males (over 60) more frequently than it does any other age group, including childhood. Myasthenia gravis is not transmissible or hereditary. On rare occasions, multiple family members may experience the illness.

It may impair ones capacity for:

- Blink or move your eyes.
- Maintain an open gaze.
- Make gestures with your face.
- Suck, chew, and speak.
- Raise your arms and pick up things.
- Move from a chair or go upstairs.
- Muscle weakness increases with exercise and

> decreases following rest. Usually, symptoms appear rapidly.
> - Chronic (long-lasting) neuromuscular disease that damages the junction between your muscles and nerves is called myasthenia gravis.

A malfunction in the transmission of nerve signals to muscles, specifically when the nerve and muscle are unable to communicate at the neuromuscular junction, is the cause of myasthenia gravis. Neurons, or brain cells, communicate with one another through substances called neurotransmitters. Acetylcholine is a neurotransmitter released by the nerve ends when electrical signals or impulses responsible for causing muscle activity pass along that nerve. The process that causes the muscle to contract is triggered when acetylcholine attaches to receptors on the muscle.

In myasthenia gravis, the immune system's generated antibodies block, modify, or eliminate acetylcholine receptors at the neuromuscular junction, preventing the muscle from contracting. The acetylcholine receptor itself is the target of most of these antibodies, although other proteins, such the MuSK (Muscle-Specific Kinase) protein, can also induce transmission impairments at the neuromuscular junction.

The immune system is regulated by the thymus gland, which may also be linked to myasthenia gravis. Up until adolescence, the thymus gland expands gradually. After that, it shrinks until fat replaces it. Since the thymus is in charge of manufacturing T-lymphocytes, also known as T cells, a particular kind of white blood cell that defends the body against viruses and illnesses, it plays a significant role in the immune system's development throughout childhood. The thymus gland persists in size in a significant number of adult myasthenia gravis patients. In addition to developing tumours in the thymus gland known as thymomas, individuals with the condition usually have clusters of immune cells in their thymus gland. Though they can develop into cancer, thymomas are usually benign. Researchers think that the immune system may attack its own cells and tissues and manufacture acetylcholine receptor antibodies as a result of the thymus gland providing growing immune cells with erroneous instructions. Rarely, a number of common drugs, such as statins, which are administered to help decrease cholesterol, can make myasthenia gravis worse. Patients suffering from myasthenia gravis should discuss any potential drug interactions with their physician.

Causes and Pathophysiology of Myasthenia Gravis

The exact causes of Myasthenia Gravis are not fully understood, but researchers have identified several factors that contribute to the development and progression of this autoimmune disorder. The pathophysiology of Myasthenia Gravis involves a complex interplay between genetic and environmental factors, leading to an abnormal immune response and disruption of neuromuscular communication.

Genetic Factors

Genetic predisposition plays a significant role in the development of Myasthenia Gravis. Certain genes, particularly those related to the human leukocyte antigen (HLA) system, have been associated with an increased risk of developing the disease. The HLA genes are responsible for regulating the immune system's ability to recognize and respond to foreign substances.

Individuals with specific HLA gene variants, such as HLA-DR3 and HLA-B8, have a higher likelihood of developing Myasthenia Gravis. These genetic variations may contribute to the abnormal recognition of acetylcholine receptors as foreign, triggering an autoimmune attack.

Environmental Factors

While genetics play a crucial role, environmental factors can also contribute to the development of Myasthenia Gravis. Potential environmental triggers include:

1. Viral infections: Certain viral infections, such as the Epstein-Barr virus (EBV), have been linked to an increased risk of developing Myasthenia Gravis. These infections may activate the immune system and lead to an

autoimmune response.

2. Medications: Some medications, such as certain antibiotics (e.g., aminoglycosides), cardiovascular drugs (e.g., quinidine), and chemotherapeutic agents, have been associated with the development of myasthenic symptoms or exacerbation of existing Myasthenia Gravis.

3. Stress: Emotional and physical stress can potentially trigger or worsen the symptoms of Myasthenia Gravis, possibly by altering the immune system's function.

4. Hormonal changes: Fluctuations in hormone levels, such as during pregnancy or menopause, may influence the disease's course and severity.

A Historical Perspective on Myasthenia Gravis

Myasthenia Gravis, a Latin term that translates to "grave muscle weakness," has a rich and intriguing history spanning centuries. The earliest known description of this condition can be traced back to the 17th century when Sir Thomas Willis, an English physician, documented cases of individuals experiencing fluctuating muscle weakness and fatigue. However, it wasn't until the late 19th century that the term "Myasthenia Gravis" was coined by German physician Wilhelm Erb, who recognized it as a distinct clinical entity characterized by a pathological state of fatigability.

Throughout the 20th century, significant advancements

were made in understanding and managing Myasthenia Gravis. In 1934, Mary Brodkey Walker and Alfred Blalock performed the first successful Thymectomy (removal of the thymus gland) on a patient with Myasthenia Gravis, leading to remarkable improvements in their condition. This discovery paved the way for further research into the role of the thymus gland in the disease's pathogenesis.

The true breakthrough came in the 1960s when Patrick Newburg-Schultz and colleagues at Yale University identified the presence of acetylcholine receptor antibodies in the blood of patients with Myasthenia Gravis. This groundbreaking discovery unveiled the autoimmune nature of the disease and laid the foundation for developing more targeted therapies. Over the decades, researchers and clinicians have relentlessly worked to unravel the complexities of Myasthenia Gravis, leading to improved diagnostic techniques, more effective treatments, and a deeper understanding of the disease's underlying mechanisms.

Research sketch

Myasthenia Gravis is a global health concern, affecting individuals across diverse populations and regions. Researchers worldwide have dedicated their efforts to understand the disease's prevalence, impact, and potential risk factors. Numerous studies have been conducted, shedding light on the far-reaching effects of this autoimmune disorder.

According to a comprehensive review published in the Journal of Neurology, Neurosurgery, and Psychiatry, the global prevalence of Myasthenia Gravis ranges from 1 to 10 cases per 100,000 individuals, with variations across different geographic regions. The disease is more common in women, particularly those of childbearing age, and the incidence tends to increase with age.

In the United States, Myasthenia Gravis is considered a rare disease, affecting approximately 20 out of every 100,000 individuals. However, its impact on quality of life and economic burden is substantial. A study conducted by the Myasthenia Gravis Foundation of America revealed that the disease significantly affects employment, with over 60% of patients reporting limitations in their ability to work or maintain employment.

In Asia, particularly in countries like Japan and China, the prevalence of Myasthenia Gravis is relatively higher compared to Western nations. Researchers attribute this to potential genetic and environmental factors influencing the disease's pathogenesis. Studies in these regions have focused on identifying potential risk factors, such as specific HLA (Human Leukocyte Antigen) gene variations and exposure to certain environmental triggers.

Research efforts have also explored the impact of Myasthenia Gravis on mental health and overall well-being. Studies have consistently reported higher rates of anxiety, depression, and reduced quality of life among patients with Myasthenia Gravis compared to the general population. This underscores the need for comprehensive care approaches that address both the physical and psychological aspects of the disease. Ongoing research initiatives aim to further elucidate the molecular mechanisms underlying Myasthenia Gravis, identify potential biomarkers for early diagnosis, and develop novel therapeutic strategies to improve patient outcomes and quality of life.

Pathophysiology

The underlying pathophysiology of Myasthenia Gravis involves an autoimmune attack on the acetylcholine receptors (AChRs) located on the postsynaptic membrane of the neuromuscular junction. This disrupts the normal communication between nerve cells and muscle cells, leading to muscle weakness and fatigue.

In most cases of Myasthenia Gravis, the immune system produces antibodies called anti-AChR antibodies, which bind to and block or destroy the acetylcholine receptors on muscle cells. This disrupts the binding of acetylcholine, the neurotransmitter responsible for triggering muscle contraction.

Additionally, in some cases, the thymus gland (an organ located in the upper chest) plays a role in the disease's pathogenesis. The thymus is involved in the development and maturation of T-cells, a type of immune cell. In Myasthenia Gravis, the thymus may be abnormal, leading to the production of self-reactive T-cells that contribute to the autoimmune attack on acetylcholine receptors. The combination of genetic predisposition, environmental triggers, and abnormal immune system activation results in a perpetuating cycle of autoimmune attack on the neuromuscular junction, leading to the characteristic muscle weakness and fatigue associated with Myasthenia Gravis.

The Role of Acetylcholine Receptor Antibodies

Acetylcholine receptor (AChR) antibodies play a crucial role in the pathogenesis of Myasthenia Gravis, as they are the primary mediators of the autoimmune attack on the neuromuscular junction. These antibodies are produced by the body's own immune system, which mistakenly recognizes the acetylcholine receptors on muscle cells as foreign entities and mounts an attack against them.

The acetylcholine receptors are proteins located on the surface of muscle cells at the neuromuscular junction. They are responsible for receiving the chemical signal (acetylcholine) released by nerve cells, which triggers muscle contraction. In Myasthenia Gravis, the presence of AChR antibodies disrupts this normal communication process, leading to muscle weakness and fatigue.

There are several mechanisms by which AChR antibodies can impair neuromuscular transmission:

1. Binding and blocking: AChR antibodies can bind to the acetylcholine receptors on muscle cells, physically blocking the binding site for acetylcholine. This prevents the neurotransmitter from initiating muscle contraction, resulting in muscle weakness.

2. Complement-mediated damage: AChR antibodies can activate the complement system, a part of the immune system responsible for destroying foreign substances. The activated complement proteins can damage and destroy the acetylcholine receptors, leading to a reduction in their number on the muscle cell surface.

3. Antigenic modulation: AChR antibodies can cross-link and cap the acetylcholine receptors, causing them to be internalized and degraded by the muscle cells. This process, known as antigenic modulation, reduces the number of available receptors for neuromuscular transmission.

4. Interference with receptor clustering: The formation of AChR antibodies can disrupt the clustering of acetylcholine receptors on the postsynaptic membrane, which is essential for efficient neuromuscular transmission.

The presence and levels of AChR antibodies in the blood are used as a diagnostic marker for Myasthenia Gravis. Patients with generalized Myasthenia Gravis typically have detectable AChR antibodies, while those with ocular Myasthenia Gravis may or may not have these antibodies.

It is important to note that not all cases of Myasthenia Gravis are associated with AChR antibodies. In some cases, the disease may be mediated by antibodies against other proteins involved in neuromuscular transmission, such as muscle-specific kinase (MuSK) or lipoprotein-related protein 4 (LRP4). These cases are referred to as seronegative Myasthenia Gravis.

Understanding the role of AChR antibodies in Myasthenia Gravis has been crucial for developing targeted therapies, such as plasmapheresis (removal of antibodies from the blood) and immunosuppressive treatments, which aim to reduce the production of these harmful antibodies and alleviate the symptoms of muscle weakness.

Types of Myasthenia Gravis

Myasthenia Gravis can manifest in different forms, depending on the extent and distribution of muscle weakness. The three main types of Myasthenia Gravis are ocular, generalized, and seronegative.

Ocular Myasthenia Gravis

Ocular Myasthenia Gravis (OMG) is characterized by muscle weakness primarily affecting the extraocular muscles, which control eye movements. Individuals with OMG may experience the following symptoms:

1. Drooping eyelids (ptosis)

2. Double vision (diplopia)

3. Difficulty with eye movements, including up/down and side-to-side movements

In OMG, the muscle weakness is typically confined to the eye region, and other muscles in the body are not affected initially. However, in some cases, OMG can progress to generalized Myasthenia Gravis over time.

Approximately 50% of individuals with OMG have detectable levels of acetylcholine receptor (AChR) antibodies in their blood, while the remaining cases are seronegative.

Generalized Myasthenia Gravis

Generalized Myasthenia Gravis (GMG) is the most common form of the disease, affecting multiple muscle groups throughout the body. In addition to the ocular symptoms seen in OMG, individuals with GMG may experience the following:

1. Weakness in the facial muscles, leading to a drooping mouth, difficulty chewing, and swallowing problems

2. Slurred speech (dysarthria)

3. Weakness in the limb muscles, making it difficult to perform activities like climbing stairs, lifting objects, or walking long

distances

4. Difficulty breathing due to weakness in the respiratory muscles

GMG can involve a wide range of skeletal muscles, and the severity of symptoms can fluctuate throughout the day or during periods of increased activity or stress.

Most individuals with GMG have detectable levels of AChR antibodies in their blood, which is a key diagnostic marker for this form of the disease.

Seronegative Myasthenia Gravis

Seronegative Myasthenia Gravis (SNMG) is a subtype of the disease in which individuals do not have detectable levels of AChR antibodies in their blood. However, they still exhibit symptoms of muscle weakness and fatigue characteristic of Myasthenia Gravis.

In SNMG, the autoimmune attack is thought to be mediated by antibodies against other proteins involved in neuromuscular transmission, such as muscle-specific kinase (MuSK) or lipoprotein-related protein 4 (LRP4). These antibodies can interfere with the proper clustering and functioning of acetylcholine receptors on the muscle cells, leading to impaired neuromuscular transmission.

SNMG can present as either ocular or generalized forms, and the symptoms are similar to those observed in AChR antibody-positive cases. However, the absence of detectable AChR antibodies can make the diagnosis more challenging, requiring additional testing and careful clinical evaluation.

Understanding the different types of Myasthenia Gravis is crucial for accurate diagnosis, treatment planning, and monitoring disease progression. Each form may require tailored therapeutic approaches and management strategies to effectively address the specific underlying mechanisms and clinical manifestations.

CHAPTER TWO

Diagnosis and Evaluation

Recognizing The Symptoms Of Myasthenia Gravis

Myasthenia Gravis (MG) is a complex autoimmune disorder that presents with a range of symptoms, primarily affecting the skeletal muscles. Early recognition of these symptoms is crucial for prompt diagnosis and effective management. The hallmark symptom of MG is fluctuating muscle weakness that worsens with activity and improves with rest. This weakness can manifest in various ways:

1. **Eye muscle weakness (Ocular Myasthenia):** Double vision (diplopia), drooping eyelids (ptosis), or difficulty focusing the eyes are often the initial symptoms experienced by many MG patients. These ocular symptoms can be intermittent or persistent and may be exacerbated by prolonged reading, watching television, or other visually demanding tasks.

2. **Facial muscle weakness**: Patients may

experience difficulty in maintaining facial expressions, leading to a "mask-like" appearance or a drooping mouth. Chewing and swallowing can also become challenging as the disease progresses.

3. **Limb muscle weakness**: As the disease advances, patients may experience weakness in the arms, legs, or neck muscles, making tasks like climbing stairs, lifting objects, or holding the head upright increasingly difficult.

4. **Respiratory muscle weakness**: In severe cases, the muscles involved in breathing can be affected, leading to shortness of breath, difficulty speaking, or even respiratory failure, which requires immediate medical attention.

It's important to note that the symptoms of MG can vary widely from person to person, and the pattern of muscle weakness can fluctuate throughout the day or even within the same day. Some patients may experience a remission of symptoms, while others may have a more progressive course.

Diagnostic Tests for Myasthenia Gravis

Diagnosing Myasthenia Gravis involves a combination of clinical examination, laboratory tests, and specialized procedures. The diagnostic process typically involves the following steps:

1. **Medical history and physical examination**:

A thorough medical history and physical examination are essential to identify symptoms and assess muscle weakness patterns. The physician may perform specific tests, such as the ice pack test or the sleep test, to observe changes in muscle strength.

2. **Blood tests**: Blood tests can detect the presence of antibodies against acetylcholine receptors (AChR) or muscle-specific kinase (MuSK), which are characteristic of MG. However, some patients may have negative blood tests (seronegative MG), requiring additional testing.

3. **Electromyography (EMG)**: EMG is a diagnostic test that measures the electrical activity of muscles. It can help distinguish MG from other neuromuscular disorders by detecting abnormalities in muscle fiber conduction.

4. **Repetitive nerve stimulation (RNS)**: RNS is a specialized technique that evaluates the ability of muscles to respond to repeated electrical stimulation. In MG patients, a decremental response (a progressive reduction in muscle contraction) is often observed.

5. **Single-fiber electromyography (SFEMG)**: SFEMG is a highly sensitive test that measures the electrical activity of individual muscle fibers. It can detect abnormalities in neuromuscular transmission, even in patients with negative antibody tests.

6. **Imaging tests**: Imaging techniques such as computed tomography (CT) or magnetic resonance imaging (MRI) may be used to assess the presence of a thymoma (a tumor of the thymus gland) or other underlying conditions that can contribute to MG.

Differentiating Myasthenia Gravis from Other Conditions

Myasthenia Gravis shares some symptoms with other neuromuscular disorders, making differential diagnosis essential. Conditions that may mimic MG include:

1. **Lambert-Eaton Myasthenic Syndrome (LEMS)**: LEMS is an autoimmune disorder that affects the neuromuscular junction, but it is typically associated with underlying malignancies, such as small cell lung cancer.

2. **Congenital Myasthenic Syndromes**: These are a group of inherited disorders that affect the neuromuscular junction and can present with similar symptoms to MG.

3. **Botulism**: Botulism is a rare but serious illness caused by a neurotoxin produced by the bacterium Clostridium botulinum, which can lead to muscle weakness and paralysis.

4. **Myopathies**: Various muscle disorders, such as muscular dystrophies or inflammatory myopathies, can cause muscle weakness and may initially resemble MG.

5. **Thyroid disorders**: Conditions like hypothyroidism or hyperthyroidism can sometimes cause muscle weakness and

fatigue, mimicking MG symptoms.

Accurate differentiation between MG and other conditions is crucial for appropriate treatment and management. A combination of clinical observations, laboratory tests, and specialized diagnostic procedures is often necessary to establish the correct diagnosis.

The Importance of Early Diagnosis

Early diagnosis of Myasthenia Gravis is crucial for several reasons:

1. **Prompt treatment initiation**: Early diagnosis allows for the timely initiation of appropriate treatment, which can help prevent further progression of the disease and potentially reduce the risk of life-threatening complications, such as respiratory failure.

2. **Better management of symptoms**: Early intervention can help manage symptoms more effectively, improving the patient's quality of life and reducing the burden of the disease.

3. **Prevention of complications**: Undiagnosed or untreated MG can lead to various complications, including respiratory distress, aspiration pneumonia, and muscle atrophy. Early diagnosis and treatment can help prevent or minimize these complications.

4. **Identification of underlying conditions**: In some cases, MG may be associated with other underlying conditions, such as thymoma

or thyroid disorders. Early diagnosis allows for the identification and appropriate management of these conditions.

5. **Psychological support**: Receiving an early diagnosis can provide patients with a better understanding of their condition and access to support resources, reducing the emotional and psychological burden associated with the uncertainty of undiagnosed symptoms.

6. **Planning and decision-making**: An early diagnosis enables patients and their families to make informed decisions about treatment options, lifestyle adjustments, and future planning, empowering them to take an active role in managing their condition.

While the diagnostic process for MG can be complex, timely recognition and evaluation are essential for optimal patient outcomes and improved quality of life.

Multidisciplinary Approach to Evaluation

Myasthenia Gravis is a complex condition that affects multiple aspects of a patient's life, necessitating a multidisciplinary approach to evaluation and management. A comprehensive care team may include the following healthcare professionals:

1. **Neurologist**: A neurologist specializing in neuromuscular disorders plays a central role in the diagnosis, treatment, and ongoing management of MG. They are responsible for interpreting diagnostic tests, prescribing

appropriate medications, and monitoring the patient's response to treatment.

2. **Ophthalmologist**: As ocular symptoms are often the first manifestation of MG, an ophthalmologist can assist in evaluating and managing eye-related issues, such as ptosis (drooping eyelids) and diplopia (double vision).

3. **Pulmonologist**: In cases where respiratory muscles are affected, a pulmonologist can evaluate and manage respiratory function, including the potential need for ventilatory support or other interventions.

4. **Physiotherapist**: A physiotherapist can develop customized exercise programs to help maintain muscle strength, improve mobility, and prevent complications associated with prolonged inactivity or weakness.

5. **Occupational therapist**: An occupational therapist can assist patients in adapting their daily activities and environment to accommodate their functional limitations, promoting independence and quality of life.

6. **Speech-language pathologist**: For patients experiencing difficulties with swallowing or speech due to weakness in the facial and throat muscles, a speech-language pathologist can provide evaluation and targeted interventions.

7. **Dietitian**: A dietitian can help develop

nutritional plans tailored to the patient's specific needs, ensuring adequate caloric and nutrient intake, especially during periods of exacerbation or difficulty swallowing.

8. **Psychologist or counselor**: Coping with a chronic condition like MG can be emotionally challenging. A psychologist or counselor can provide invaluable support, helping patients and their families manage stress, anxiety, and depression associated with the disease.

9. **Social worker**: Social workers can assist patients and their families in navigating complex healthcare systems, accessing community resources, and addressing any financial or social concerns related to their condition.

Collaboration among this multidisciplinary team is essential for delivering comprehensive and coordinated care that addresses the various aspects of Myasthenia Gravis. Regular communication and care coordination ensure that the patient's needs are met holistically, promoting better disease management and overall well-being.

CHAPTER THREE

*Living with Ocular
Myasthenia Gravis*

Ocular Myasthenia Gravis (OMG) is a distinct form of Myasthenia Gravis (MG), a chronic autoimmune disorder that primarily affects the muscles responsible for eye movements and facial expressions. In this condition, the body's immune system mistakenly attacks and weakens the neuromuscular junction, leading to impaired communication between nerves and muscles. OMG is characterized by the isolated involvement of the extraocular muscles, which control eye movements, and sometimes the levator palpebrae superioris muscle, responsible for eyelid elevation. This localized form of MG can significantly impact an individual's quality of life, as the eyes play a crucial role in daily activities and social interactions.

Symptoms and Diagnosis of Ocular Myasthenia Gravis

The hallmark symptom of OMG is fluctuating double vision (diplopia), which can worsen with prolonged use of the eyes or as the day progresses. Patients may also experience drooping eyelids (ptosis), which can affect one or both eyes and vary in severity throughout the day.

Other common symptoms of OMG include:

- Blurred vision
- Difficulty focusing
- Eye strain and fatigue
- Sensitivity to bright lights

Diagnosing OMG can be challenging, as the symptoms may be intermittent and can mimic other neurological or ophthalmological conditions. A comprehensive evaluation by a neurologist or ophthalmologist is essential, which may include:

- A detailed medical history and physical examination
- Blood tests to detect acetylcholine receptor (AChR) antibodies
- Specialized tests like the ice pack test, sleep test, or edrophonium (Tensilon) test
- Imaging studies (CT or MRI) to evaluate the thymus gland

Early and accurate diagnosis is crucial for prompt treatment and management of OMG.

Treatment Options for Ocular Myasthenia Gravis

The treatment approach for OMG aims to alleviate symptoms, improve muscle strength, and prevent potential progression to generalized Myasthenia Gravis. Several treatment options are available, including:

1. Acetylcholinesterase inhibitors (e.g., pyridostigmine): These medications help prolong the action of acetylcholine at the neuromuscular junction, improving muscle function.

2. Immunosuppressant drugs (e.g., corticosteroids, azathioprine, mycophenolate mofetil): These medications are used to suppress the autoimmune response and reduce antibody production.

3. Intravenous immunoglobulin (IVIG) or plasma exchange (PLEX): These therapies can quickly improve symptoms during acute exacerbations or crises by removing harmful antibodies or providing temporary replacement of antibodies.

4. Thymectomy (surgical removal of the thymus gland): This procedure may be recommended in certain cases, as the thymus gland is believed to play a role in the development of MG.

The choice of treatment depends on factors such as the severity of symptoms, the patient's age, overall health, and response to previous treatments.

Managing Daily Life with Ocular Myasthenia Gravis

Living with OMG can be challenging, but with proper management and lifestyle modifications, individuals can maintain a good quality of life. Some strategies to consider include:

- Identifying and avoiding potential triggers, such as stress, fatigue, and extreme temperatures
- Incorporating rest periods throughout the day to minimize eye strain
- Using adaptive equipment or assistive devices (e.g., prism glasses, eye patches) to improve vision and reduce double vision
- Seeking support from occupational therapists, counselors, or support groups to address practical and emotional challenges
- Maintaining a balanced diet and engaging in regular, low-impact exercise to promote overall well-being

Potential Progression to Generalized Myasthenia Gravis

While OMG is initially limited to the eye muscles, it is important to be aware of the potential progression to generalized Myasthenia Gravis (GMG). In some cases, the autoimmune process can spread to other muscle groups, leading to more widespread weakness and additional symptoms.

The risk of progression to GMG varies among individuals and can be influenced by factors such as age, gender, and the presence of certain antibodies. Regular monitoring by a neurologist and prompt treatment are crucial to manage any potential progression and prevent life-threatening complications.

It is essential for individuals with OMG to be vigilant about any new or worsening symptoms and to report them to their healthcare provider immediately. Early intervention and appropriate management can greatly improve the prognosis and quality of life for those living with Myasthenia Gravis.

CHAPTER FOUR

*Coping with Generalized
Myasthenia Gravis*

What Is Generalized Myasthenia Gravis?

Generalized Myasthenia Gravis (GMG) is a severe form of the autoimmune disorder Myasthenia Gravis, in which the body's immune system mistakenly attacks and weakens multiple muscle groups throughout the body. Unlike the ocular form, which primarily affects the eye muscles, GMG impacts various skeletal muscles, leading to widespread muscular weakness and fatigue. In GMG, the immune system produces antibodies that disrupt the normal transmission of signals from nerves to muscles, impairing the ability of muscles to contract and function properly. This disruption can affect muscles involved in essential functions like breathing, swallowing, and movement.

Symptoms and Diagnosis of Generalized
Myasthenia Gravis

The symptoms of GMG can vary in severity and distribution, but they typically involve muscle weakness and fatigue that worsen with prolonged activity and improve with rest. Common symptoms include:

1. Generalized muscle weakness: Patients may experience weakness in the arms, legs, neck, and trunk muscles, making daily activities increasingly challenging.

2. Difficulty swallowing (dysphagia): Weakness in the muscles involved in swallowing can lead to choking, coughing, or aspirating food and liquids.

3. Difficulty breathing: Weakness in the respiratory muscles can cause shortness of breath, particularly after exertion or lying down.

4. Facial muscle weakness: Patients may experience drooping eyelids (ptosis), difficulty smiling or chewing, and a slurred speech pattern.

5. Fatigue: Persistent muscle weakness and the effort required to perform daily tasks can lead to extreme fatigue.

Diagnosing GMG typically involves a combination of clinical examinations, blood tests to detect specific antibodies, and electrodiagnostic tests such as repetitive nerve stimulation or single-fiber electromyography.

Treatment Approaches for Generalized Myasthenia Gravis

The treatment of GMG aims to manage symptoms, improve muscle strength, and prevent potentially life-threatening complications. Common treatment approaches include:

1. Medications: Cholinesterase inhibitors like pyridostigmine are typically the first line of treatment, as they improve neuromuscular transmission and enhance muscle strength. Immunosuppressant drugs like corticosteroids, azathioprine, or mycophenolate mofetil may also be prescribed to modulate the immune system's response.

2. Intravenous immunoglobulin (IVIG) or plasma exchange (PLEX): These treatments can rapidly remove or neutralize the harmful antibodies, providing temporary relief during severe exacerbations or crisis situations.

3. Thymectomy: Surgical removal of the thymus gland, which plays a role in the development of Myasthenia Gravis, can lead to long-term improvement or potential remission in some patients.

4. Supportive therapies: Physical therapy, occupational therapy, and speech therapy can help patients maintain muscle function, improve activities of daily living, and manage swallowing difficulties.

Managing Exacerbations and Crisis Situations

Patients with GMG may experience periods of worsening

symptoms, known as exacerbations or myasthenic crises. These situations can be life-threatening if not addressed promptly and may require hospitalization and intensive care. Prompt recognition and management of these episodes are crucial.

Exacerbations can be triggered by various factors, including infections, stress, certain medications, or underlying health conditions. During these episodes, patients may experience severe muscle weakness, difficulty swallowing or breathing, and an increased risk of respiratory failure.

Crisis management may involve:

1. Intravenous immunoglobulin (IVIG) or plasma exchange (PLEX) to rapidly remove harmful antibodies.

2. Ventilatory support: In severe cases, patients may require mechanical ventilation to assist with breathing.

3. Intensive monitoring and supportive care in an intensive care unit (ICU) setting.

Lifestyle Adjustments for Generalized Myasthenia Gravis

Living with GMG often requires making lifestyle adjustments to manage symptoms, conserve energy, and maintain overall well-being. These adjustments may include:

1. Pacing activities: Breaking up tasks into smaller, more manageable steps and allowing

for rest periods can help prevent excessive fatigue and muscle weakness.

2. Dietary modifications: Avoiding foods that exacerbate muscle weakness, such as those high in salt or sugar, and maintaining a balanced diet can aid in symptom management.

3. Exercise and physical activity: Engaging in low-impact exercises like walking, swimming, or gentle stretching can help maintain muscle strength and overall fitness, while avoiding overexertion.

4. Assistive devices: Using mobility aids like canes, walkers, or wheelchairs can help conserve energy and prevent falls.

5. Stress management: Incorporating relaxation techniques, such as deep breathing exercises or meditation, can help reduce stress and its impact on symptoms.

6. Support systems: Building a support network of family, friends, and healthcare professionals can provide emotional support and practical assistance when needed.

CHAPTER FIVE

*Understanding Seronegative
Myasthenia Gravis*

Seronegative Myasthenia Gravis (SNMG) is a rare and distinct form of Myasthenia Gravis (MG), a chronic autoimmune neuromuscular disorder characterized by fluctuating muscle weakness. In this variant, patients exhibit clinical symptoms of MG, but their blood tests fail to detect the presence of acetylcholine receptor (AChR) antibodies, the primary autoantibodies associated with the more common forms of MG. While the exact underlying mechanisms of SNMG are not fully understood, researchers believe that other autoantibodies or immune system factors may be involved in disrupting the normal function of the neuromuscular junction, leading to muscle weakness and fatigue. This enigmatic form of MG poses unique challenges in diagnosis and management, as the absence of the well-known AChR antibodies can make it more difficult to identify and treat effectively.

Diagnosis and Testing for Seronegative

Myasthenia Gravis

Diagnosing SNMG can be a complex and multifaceted process, as it relies on a combination of clinical evaluation, specialized testing, and ruling out other potential causes of muscle weakness. Several diagnostic approaches may be employed:

1. **Clinical Evaluation**: A thorough medical history and physical examination are crucial in assessing the pattern and distribution of muscle weakness, as well as its fluctuating nature. Physicians may also administer tests such as the ice pack test or the Tensilon (edrophonium) test to observe the temporary improvement or worsening of symptoms.

2. **Antibody Testing**: While AChR antibodies are absent in SNMG patients, other autoantibodies, such as those against muscle-specific kinase (MuSK) or lipoprotein-related protein 4 (LRP4), may be detected through specialized blood tests.

3. **Electrophysiological Studies**: Electromyography (EMG) and repetitive nerve stimulation tests can provide valuable insights into the function of the neuromuscular junction and help support a diagnosis of SNMG.

4. **Imaging Techniques**: Chest computed tomography (CT) scans or magnetic resonance imaging (MRI) may be performed to rule out the presence of thymomas or other

underlying conditions that could contribute to muscle weakness.

5. **Therapeutic Trial**: In some cases, physicians may initiate a trial of acetylcholinesterase inhibitors or other MG treatments to observe the patient's response, which can aid in confirming or ruling out a diagnosis of SNMG.

Treatment Options for Seronegative Myasthenia Gravis

While the treatment approach for SNMG shares similarities with other forms of MG, the lack of specific antibody targets can make it more challenging to manage. Common treatment strategies include:

1. **Acetylcholinesterase Inhibitors**: Medications like pyridostigmine or neostigmine can help improve muscle strength by prolonging the action of acetylcholine at the neuromuscular junction.

2. **Immunosuppressive Therapies**: Corticosteroids, such as prednisone, or other immunosuppressive drugs may be prescribed to modulate the overactive immune response and reduce muscle weakness.

3. **Intravenous Immunoglobulin (IVIG)** or **Plasma Exchange (PLEX)**: These therapies aim to remove circulating autoantibodies or provide temporary relief from symptoms during acute exacerbations or myasthenic crises.

4. **Thymectomy**: In some cases, surgical removal of the thymus gland may be

considered, even in the absence of a thymoma, as it has been shown to improve symptoms in certain SNMG patients.

5. **Supportive Care**: Physical therapy, occupational therapy, and assistive devices may be recommended to help manage daily activities and improve quality of life.

Challenges in Managing Seronegative Myasthenia Gravis

Despite the available treatment options, managing SNMG can be particularly challenging due to several factors:

1. **Lack of Specific Antibody Targets**: Without a clear understanding of the underlying autoantibodies or immune mechanisms, targeted therapies may be less effective.

2. **Variable Response to Treatments**: Patients with SNMG may respond differently to standard MG treatments, making it difficult to predict therapeutic outcomes and optimize management strategies.

3. **Fluctuating Symptoms**: The unpredictable nature of symptom fluctuations can make it challenging to adjust treatment regimens and maintain consistent symptom control.

4. **Potential Misdiagnosis**: The absence of AChR antibodies and the rarity of SNMG can lead to misdiagnosis or delayed diagnosis, further complicating treatment initiation and disease management.

Ongoing Research and Future Perspectives

Researchers are actively investigating the underlying mechanisms and potential autoantibody targets in SNMG, with the goal of developing more targeted and effective treatments. Several areas of ongoing research include:

1. **Identification of Novel Autoantibodies**: Advances in immunology and proteomic techniques may lead to the discovery of new autoantibodies associated with SNMG, providing insights into disease pathogenesis and potential therapeutic targets.

2. **Exploring Genetic Factors**: Genetic studies may uncover predisposing genetic variants or mutations that contribute to the development of SNMG, potentially leading to personalized treatment approaches.

3. **Clinical Trials**: New experimental therapies, such as monoclonal antibodies or targeted immunotherapies, are being evaluated in clinical trials for their potential to improve outcomes in SNMG patients.

4. **Biomarker Development**: Identifying reliable biomarkers specific to SNMG could aid in earlier diagnosis, monitoring disease progression, and assessing treatment response.

5. **Patient-Centered Research**: Ongoing research efforts aim to better understand the impact of SNMG on patients' quality of life, addressing their specific needs and

developing comprehensive care strategies.

As our understanding of SNMG continues to evolve, there is hope for improved diagnostic methods, more targeted therapies, and enhanced management strategies that will ultimately lead to better outcomes and improved quality of life for individuals affected by this rare and challenging form of Myasthenia Gravis.

CHAPTER SIX

*Medical Management
and Treatments*

Pharmacological Treatments For Myasthenia Gravis

Myasthenia Gravis (MG) is a chronic autoimmune disorder that affects the neuromuscular junctions, leading to muscle weakness and fatigue. Various pharmacological treatments have been developed to manage its symptoms effectively. These medications aim to improve muscle strength, alleviate fatigue, and enhance overall quality of life for individuals living with MG.

Anticholinesterase Agents: Pyridostigmine Bromide (Mestinon) is a widely prescribed medication for MG patients. It belongs to the class of anticholinesterase agents, which work by inhibiting the enzyme acetylcholinesterase. By doing so, they prolong the availability of acetylcholine, the neurotransmitter responsible for enabling muscle contractions. This leads to improved muscle strength and reduced muscle weakness associated with MG.

Immunosuppressive Drugs: Myasthenia Gravis is an autoimmune disease, and immunosuppressive drugs play a crucial role in managing its symptoms. These medications work by suppressing the overactive immune system, reducing the production of antibodies that attack the body's own tissues. Commonly prescribed immunosuppressive drugs for MG include corticosteroids (such as prednisone), azathioprine, mycophenolate mofetil, and cyclosporine.

Intravenous Immunoglobulin (IVIG): IVIG therapy involves administering a concentrated solution of pooled human immunoglobulins intravenously. This treatment can help modulate the immune system and reduce the production of harmful antibodies in MG patients. IVIG is often used as a short-term treatment option to manage acute exacerbations or crisis situations.

Monoclonal Antibodies: Monoclonal antibodies are a newer class of medications that selectively target specific components of the immune system. Drugs like rituximab and eculizumab have shown promising results in treating certain forms of MG by depleting or inhibiting the activity of harmful immune cells or complement proteins.

Pyridostigmine Bromide and Other

Mainstream Medications

Pyridostigmine Bromide (Mestinon) is considered the mainstay of pharmacological treatment for Myasthenia Gravis. This medication belongs to the class of anticholinesterase agents and is typically the first line of treatment for managing MG symptoms. Pyridostigmine Bromide works by inhibiting the enzyme acetylcholinesterase, which is responsible for breaking down acetylcholine, the neurotransmitter that facilitates muscle contraction. By inhibiting this enzyme, Pyridostigmine Bromide allows acetylcholine to remain active for a longer period, thereby improving muscle strength and reducing muscle weakness associated with MG.

Other mainstream medications used in the treatment of Myasthenia Gravis include:

1. Corticosteroids (e.g., prednisone): These immunosuppressive drugs are often prescribed to suppress the overactive immune system and reduce the production of harmful antibodies in MG patients.

2. Azathioprine: An immunosuppressive drug that works by inhibiting the proliferation of certain immune cells, reducing the autoimmune response in MG.

3. Mycophenolate mofetil: Another immunosuppressive agent that suppresses the production of antibodies and prevents the

> proliferation of immune cells involved in the autoimmune process.
>
> 4. Cyclosporine: This immunosuppressive medication inhibits the activity of T-cells, which play a crucial role in the autoimmune response in MG.

It's important to note that while these medications can effectively manage MG symptoms, they may also have potential side effects. Close monitoring by a healthcare professional and regular follow-ups are essential to ensure the optimal dosage and minimize any adverse effects.

Unconventional and Complementary Therapies

While conventional pharmacological treatments are the mainstay for managing Myasthenia Gravis (MG), some patients may explore unconventional and complementary therapies to further alleviate their symptoms and improve their overall well-being. It is crucial to discuss these options with a healthcare professional and ensure they do not interfere with prescribed medications or exacerbate the condition.

Dietary Supplements: Certain dietary supplements may help support the body's immune system and reduce inflammation associated with MG. These include:

> 1. Vitamin D: Some studies suggest that vitamin D deficiency may be linked to an increased risk of autoimmune diseases like MG. Supplementation may help modulate

the immune system and reduce muscle weakness.

2. Omega-3 Fatty Acids: These anti-inflammatory compounds found in fish oil and certain plant sources may help reduce inflammation and autoimmune activity associated with MG.

3. Probiotics: Maintaining a healthy gut microbiome through probiotic supplementation may help regulate the immune system and alleviate some MG symptoms.

Herbal Remedies: While limited research exists, some herbal remedies are believed to have potential benefits for MG patients:

1. Curcumin (from turmeric): Known for its anti-inflammatory and antioxidant properties, curcumin may help modulate the immune system and reduce muscle weakness in some cases.

2. Green Tea: Rich in antioxidants, green tea may offer anti-inflammatory benefits and support immune function in MG patients.

3. Ginseng: This adaptogenic herb is thought to have immunomodulatory effects and may help alleviate fatigue and improve overall well-being.

Mind-Body Therapies: Incorporating mind-body practices into an MG management plan may help reduce stress, promote relaxation, and improve overall quality of life:

1. Yoga and Meditation: Gentle yoga and meditation practices can help manage stress, reduce anxiety, and improve mental well-being.

2. Acupuncture: Some MG patients report benefits from acupuncture in reducing muscle weakness, fatigue, and pain associated with the condition.

3. Massage Therapy: Therapeutic massage may help alleviate muscle tension and promote relaxation in MG patients.

It is essential to consult with a healthcare professional before incorporating any unconventional or complementary therapies into an existing treatment plan for Myasthenia Gravis.

Individualized Medication Management

Myasthenia Gravis (MG) is a complex autoimmune disorder that affects individuals in varying ways. While certain medications are commonly prescribed for managing MG symptoms, the reality is that an individualized approach to medication management is often necessary to achieve optimal results. One of the key factors in individualized medication management is the recognition that MG is a heterogeneous condition. Patients may present with different subtypes of MG, such as ocular, generalized, or seronegative forms, each with its own unique characteristics and treatment considerations.

In addition, the severity of symptoms, age, overall health status, and co-existing medical conditions can influence the choice and dosage of medications for each individual patient. For example, older adults or those with renal or hepatic impairment may require lower doses or alternative medications to minimize potential side effects. Another important aspect of individualized medication management is the consideration of potential drug interactions. MG patients may be taking multiple medications for their condition, as well as for other co-existing health issues. It is essential to carefully review and monitor all prescribed medications to ensure they do not interact in a way that could exacerbate MG symptoms or cause adverse effects.

The Role of Thymectomy and Thymomas

Thymectomy, the surgical removal of the thymus gland, is often recommended for Myasthenia Gravis (MG) patients who have a thymoma, a tumor originating from the thymic cells. Thymomas are associated with an increased production of acetylcholine receptor antibodies, which contribute to the development and progression of MG symptoms.

In patients with thymomas, thymectomy serves two primary purposes:

1. Removal of the tumor: Thymomas can be

benign or malignant, and their surgical removal is essential to prevent potential complications and the spread of cancerous cells.

2. Improvement of MG symptoms: By removing the thymus gland, the source of autoantibody production is eliminated or reduced, leading to the potential improvement or remission of MG symptoms in many patients.

However, thymectomy is not limited to MG patients with thymomas. It is also considered a treatment option for certain subgroups of MG patients without thymomas, particularly those with an early onset of generalized MG symptoms (before the age of 60) and the presence of acetylcholine receptor antibodies. The decision to undergo thymectomy is made on a case-by-case basis, considering factors such as the patient's age, severity of symptoms, and the presence or absence of thymomas or other thymic abnormalities. In general, younger patients with generalized MG and positive acetylcholine receptor antibodies are more likely to benefit from thymectomy. The procedure itself can be performed through various surgical approaches, including open thoracotomy, minimally invasive techniques like video-assisted thoracoscopic surgery (VATS), or robotic-assisted surgery. The choice of approach depends on factors such as the surgeon's expertise, the patient's overall health, and the size and location of any thymic abnormalities.

While thymectomy has been shown to improve or induce remission of MG symptoms in a significant proportion of patients, it is important to note that the procedure is not a cure for MG. Patients may still require ongoing medical management with medications and other supportive therapies to control residual symptoms or potential relapses.

CHAPTER SEVEN

*Lifestyle Strategies and
Myasthenia Gravis Nutrition*

Lifestyle Strategies For Managing Myasthenia Gravis

Adopting a well-balanced and nutrient-rich diet can play a pivotal role in managing the symptoms of Myasthenia Gravis (MG) and enhancing overall well-being. Proper nutrition not only supports muscle function but also bolsters the immune system, which is crucial for individuals with this autoimmune disorder.

Focus on lean proteins: Lean proteins are essential for rebuilding and maintaining muscle mass, which can be compromised by MG. Incorporate sources such as skinless poultry, fish, legumes, and lean cuts of meat into your diet. These proteins provide the necessary building blocks for muscle repair and growth.

Embrace whole grains: Whole grains are a rich source of complex carbohydrates, fiber, and essential vitamins and minerals. They provide sustained energy and support digestion, which can be beneficial for individuals with MG. Choose options like quinoa, brown rice, oats, and whole-grain breads and pastas.

Load up on fruits and vegetables: Fruits and vegetables are packed with antioxidants, vitamins, and minerals that support immune function and overall health. Aim for a variety of colorful produce to ensure a diverse intake of nutrients. Consider incorporating leafy greens, berries, citrus fruits, and cruciferous vegetables into your meals and snacks.

Stay hydrated: Adequate hydration is crucial for maintaining muscle function and overall health. Drink plenty of water throughout the day and incorporate hydrating beverages like herbal teas and infused waters with fruits or herbs.

Consider gut-friendly foods: Emerging research suggests a potential link between gut health and autoimmune conditions. Incorporating probiotic-rich foods like yogurt, kefir, sauerkraut, and fermented vegetables may support a healthy gut microbiome and potentially aid in managing MG symptoms.

Physical Therapy and Exercise Guidelines

Regular physical activity and exercise can help maintain muscle strength, flexibility, and overall fitness, which are essential for managing MG. However, it's crucial to approach exercise with caution and under the guidance of a qualified healthcare professional.

Low-impact aerobic exercises: Engage in low-impact aerobic activities like walking, swimming, or stationary cycling to improve cardiovascular health and overall endurance. These exercises can be adjusted based on your energy levels and muscle strength.

Resistance training: Incorporate resistance exercises, such as light weight training or resistance bands, to help maintain and improve muscle strength. Start with lower weights and gradually increase as tolerated, always prioritizing proper form and technique.

Stretching and flexibility exercises: Regular stretching and flexibility exercises can help maintain range of motion and prevent muscle tightness, which can exacerbate MG symptoms. Incorporate gentle yoga or stretching routines into your daily routine.

Pacing and rest: Listen to your body and respect its limits. Fatigue is a common symptom of MG, so it's essential to pace yourself and allow for adequate rest periods between exercises or activities.

Stress Management and Self-Care Practices

Managing stress and practicing self-care can significantly improve overall well-being and potentially alleviate some of the symptoms associated with MG.

Mindfulness and relaxation techniques: Incorporate

practices like deep breathing exercises, meditation, or progressive muscle relaxation into your daily routine. These techniques can help reduce stress, promote relaxation, and enhance overall mental well-being.

Support system: Surround yourself with a supportive network of family, friends, or a local support group. Sharing your experiences and seeking emotional support can be invaluable in coping with the challenges of living with MG.

Adequate rest and sleep: Prioritize getting enough restful sleep and practicing good sleep hygiene. Fatigue is a common symptom of MG, and adequate rest can help manage this symptom and promote overall physical and mental well-being.

Engage in enjoyable activities: Identify activities that bring you joy, relaxation, or a sense of accomplishment. Engaging in hobbies, creative pursuits, or spending time in nature can provide a much-needed respite from the daily challenges of managing MG.

Medications to Avoid for Myasthenia Gravis Patients

Certain medications can potentially exacerbate or worsen the symptoms of MG. It's crucial to consult with your healthcare provider and be vigilant about the medications you take, both prescription and over-the-counter.

Aminoglycoside antibiotics: Medications like

gentamicin, tobramycin, and neomycin can potentially worsen muscle weakness in individuals with MG. These antibiotics should be avoided unless absolutely necessary and under close medical supervision.

Certain anesthetic agents: Certain anesthetic agents, such as succinylcholine and mivacurium, can interfere with neuromuscular function and potentially trigger a myasthenic crisis. Inform your healthcare providers about your MG diagnosis before any surgical procedures.

Quinine: Quinine, often used to treat malaria or leg cramps, can exacerbate muscle weakness in individuals with MG and should be avoided.

Beta-blockers: Some beta-blocker medications, commonly used for high blood pressure or heart conditions, have been known to worsen MG symptoms in some patients. Consult with your healthcare provider for alternative options.

Statins: While statins are commonly prescribed for managing cholesterol levels, they may potentially worsen MG symptoms in some individuals. Your healthcare provider can guide you on the appropriate course of action.

Myasthenia Gravis Dietary Recommendations

Living with Myasthenia Gravis (MG) requires a comprehensive approach that combines medical treatment with a well-balanced diet. Proper nutrition plays a crucial role in managing the symptoms and promoting overall well-being. Here are some dietary recommendations for individuals with MG:

1. Emphasize lean protein sources: Lean proteins are essential for building and maintaining muscle strength, which is vital for managing MG. Choose options like grilled or baked chicken, turkey, fish, eggs, and legumes.

2. Incorporate whole grains: Whole grains provide complex carbohydrates, fiber, and essential vitamins and minerals. They help maintain energy levels and support a healthy digestive system. Opt for brown rice, quinoa, whole-wheat bread, and oats.

3. Focus on colorful fruits and vegetables: Fresh fruits and vegetables are rich in antioxidants, vitamins, and minerals that support immune function and reduce inflammation. Aim for a variety of colors to ensure a diverse range of nutrients.

4. Stay hydrated: Adequate hydration is essential for muscle function and overall health. Drink plenty of water, herbal teas, or infused waters throughout the day.

5. Limit processed foods and saturated fats: Processed foods and foods high in saturated

fats can contribute to inflammation and potentially exacerbate MG symptoms. Opt for whole, nutrient-dense foods whenever possible.

6. Incorporate sources of probiotics: Probiotics support a healthy gut microbiome, which can positively impact immune function and reduce inflammation. Include fermented foods like yogurt, kefir, sauerkraut, and kimchi in your diet.

7. Consider anti-inflammatory herbs and spices: Certain herbs and spices, such as turmeric, ginger, and garlic, have anti-inflammatory properties that may help alleviate MG symptoms.

While there is no specific diet that can cure Myasthenia Gravis (MG), a well-balanced and nutrient-dense diet can help manage symptoms, reduce inflammation, and promote overall well-being. Here are some diet recipes and foods that can be beneficial for individuals with MG:

1. Grilled Salmon with Quinoa and Roasted Vegetables:

   - Salmon is a rich source of omega-3 fatty acids, which have anti-inflammatory properties.

   - Quinoa is a whole grain that provides fiber, protein, and essential nutrients.

   - Roasted vegetables like bell peppers, zucchini, and carrots are packed with antioxidants and vitamins.

2. Spinach and Strawberry Salad with Grilled Chicken:

   - Spinach is a nutrient-dense leafy green packed with vitamins and minerals.
   - Strawberries are rich in vitamin C and have anti-inflammatory properties.
   - Grilled chicken provides lean protein essential for muscle strength.

3. Lentil and Sweet Potato Stew:

   - Lentils are a great source of plant-based protein, fiber, and iron.
   - Sweet potatoes are rich in vitamins A and C, as well as antioxidants.
   - The stew can be seasoned with anti-inflammatory herbs and spices like turmeric and ginger.

4. Greek Yogurt Parfait with Mixed Berries and Nuts:

   - Greek yogurt provides probiotics to support a healthy gut and immune system.
   - Mixed berries are packed with antioxidants and fiber.
   - Nuts like almonds and walnuts offer healthy fats and protein.

5. Baked Cod with Lemon and Herb Sauce, Served with Brown Rice and Roasted Brussels Sprouts:

   - Cod is a lean source of protein and low in saturated fat.

   - Lemon and herbs like dill and parsley add flavor without unnecessary sodium or fat.

   - Brown rice and Brussels sprouts provide complex carbohydrates, fiber, and essential nutrients.

6. Vegetable and Tofu Stir-Fry with Brown Rice:

   - Tofu is a plant-based protein source that is easy to digest.

   - Stir-frying vegetables like broccoli, bell peppers, and carrots retains their nutrient content.

   - Brown rice offers whole grains and fiber.

Remember, it's essential to consult with a healthcare professional or a registered dietitian to develop a personalized dietary plan that addresses your specific needs, preferences, and any potential nutrient deficiencies or interactions with medications.

Foods to eat and avoid while treating Myasthenia Gravis

When managing Myasthenia Gravis (MG), making informed dietary choices can significantly impact symptom management and overall well-being. Here are some foods to eat and avoid while treating MG:

Foods to eat:

1. Lean proteins: Opt for lean sources of protein like skinless poultry, fish, eggs, legumes, and lean cuts of meat. Protein is essential for building and maintaining muscle strength.

2. Whole grains: Choose whole grains such as quinoa, brown rice, whole-wheat bread, and oats. They provide complex carbohydrates, fiber, and essential nutrients.

3. Colorful fruits and vegetables: Incorporate a variety of fresh fruits and vegetables into your diet. They are rich in antioxidants, vitamins, and minerals that support immune function and reduce inflammation.

4. Healthy fats: Include sources of healthy fats like avocados, nuts, seeds, and olive oil. They provide essential fatty acids and can help reduce inflammation.

5. Probiotic-rich foods: Incorporate fermented foods like yogurt, kefir, sauerkraut, and kimchi to support a healthy gut microbiome and immune function.

6. Anti-inflammatory herbs and spices: Turmeric, ginger, garlic, and other herbs and spices can help reduce inflammation and support overall health.

Foods to avoid:

1. Processed and fried foods: Limit or

avoid processed and fried foods, as they can contribute to inflammation and may exacerbate MG symptoms.

2. Saturated and trans fats: Minimize your intake of foods high in saturated and trans fats, such as butter, margarine, and processed snacks.

3. Refined carbohydrates: Limit your consumption of refined carbohydrates like white bread, pastries, and sugary drinks, as they can spike blood sugar levels and contribute to inflammation.

4. Alcohol: Alcohol can interfere with medication and exacerbate muscle weakness in individuals with MG. It's best to avoid or limit alcohol consumption.

5. Caffeine and nicotine: Excessive caffeine and nicotine can contribute to muscle weakness and fatigue, so it's advisable to limit or avoid them.

Remember, every individual's dietary needs may vary, so it's important to consult with a healthcare professional or a registered dietitian to develop a personalized plan tailored to your specific needs and medical condition.

Myasthenia Gravis meal planning

Meal planning can be a valuable tool for individuals with Myasthenia Gravis (MG) to ensure they are consuming a well-balanced and nutrient-dense diet. This meal plan incorporates a variety of lean proteins, whole grains, fruits, vegetables, and healthy fats to support the dietary needs of individuals with Myasthenia Gravis. Remember to adjust portions and ingredients based on your personal preferences and dietary requirements. We have prepared a 14-day meal plan sample that incorporates MG-friendly foods and recipes:

Day	Breakfast	Lunch	Dinner
1	Greek yogurt parfait with mixed berries and nuts	Grilled chicken salad with mixed greens, avocado, and balsamic vinaigrette	Baked salmon with quinoa and roasted vegetables
2	Overnight oats with almond milk, chia seeds, and fresh fruit	Lentil and sweet potato stew	Grilled turkey burgers with whole-wheat buns and roasted sweet potato fries
3	Spinach and feta omelet with whole-grain toast	Tuna salad on a bed of mixed greens and whole-wheat crackers	Vegetable and tofu stir-fry with brown rice
4	Avocado toast on whole-grain bread with a side of fresh fruit	Grilled chicken Caesar salad	Baked cod with lemon and herb sauce, served with brown rice and roasted Brussels sprouts
5	Smoothie bowl with mixed berries, spinach, Greek yogurt, and chia seeds	Quinoa and black bean salad	Grilled salmon and asparagus salad with lemon vinaigrette
6	Greek yogurt with mixed berries and granola	Mediterranean chickpea salad	Baked sweet potato with spinach and feta
7	Avocado and egg toast	Lentil and vegetable soup	Grilled chicken and vegetable skewers
8	Overnight oats with almond milk and fresh fruit	Tuna and white bean salad	Quinoa and roasted vegetable bowl
9	Spinach and feta frittata	Grilled chicken and vegetable wraps	Lentil and sweet potato shepherd's pie
10	Smoothie bowl with mixed berries,	Greek salad with grilled shrimp	Baked salmon with mango salsa

	spinach, and Greek yogurt		
11	Greek yogurt parfait with mixed berries and nuts	Quinoa and black bean burrito bowls	Grilled portobello mushroom caps with spinach and feta
12	Whole-grain toast with avocado and a side of fresh fruit	Roasted vegetable and hummus sandwich	Vegetable and lentil curry
13	Spinach and feta omelet with whole-grain toast	Quinoa and roasted vegetable stuffed bell peppers	Baked salmon with pesto and roasted potatoes
14	Overnight oats with almond milk, chia seeds, and fresh fruit	Grilled chicken and pineapple skewers	Lentil and sweet potato shepherd's pie

CHAPTER EIGHT

Myasthenia Gravis Diet Recipes

Grilled Salmon with Quinoa and Roasted Vegetables

Ingredients:

- 4 salmon fillets (about 6 oz each)
- 1 cup uncooked quinoa
- 2 bell peppers (any color), sliced
- 1 zucchini, sliced into rounds
- 2 carrots, peeled and sliced diagonally
- 1/4 cup olive oil
- 1 lemon, juiced
- Salt and freshly ground black pepper, to taste

Step-by-Step Preparation Instructions:

1. Preheat your grill to medium-high heat and lightly oil the grates.

2. Rinse the quinoa under cold water and place it in a saucepan with 2 cups of water. Bring to a boil, then reduce heat to low, cover, and simmer for 15-20 minutes, or until the quinoa is fluffy and the water is absorbed.

3. In a large bowl, toss the sliced bell peppers, zucchini, and carrots with 2 tablespoons of

olive oil, salt, and pepper.

4. Arrange the seasoned vegetables on a baking sheet and roast in the preheated oven or grill for about 15-20 minutes, or until tender and slightly charred, tossing occasionally.

5. While the vegetables are roasting, brush the salmon fillets with the remaining 2 tablespoons of olive oil and season with salt, pepper, and lemon juice.

6. Grill the salmon fillets for about 4-5 minutes per side, or until cooked through and the flesh flakes easily with a fork.

7. Fluff the cooked quinoa with a fork and transfer it to a serving platter or individual plates.

8. Arrange the grilled salmon and roasted vegetables over the quinoa.

9. Garnish with fresh lemon wedges and chopped fresh parsley or cilantro, if desired.

Nutritional Information (per serving):

- Calories: 450
- Protein: 35g
- Carbohydrates: 30g
- Fiber: 5g
- Fat: 20g

Dietary Recommendation

For people who are eating a diet rich in nutrients and well-balanced, this dish is a great option. It's a well-rounded and filling dinner because of the lean protein from the salmon, the complex carbohydrates from the quinoa, and the variety of vitamins and minerals from the roasted veggies.

A strong supply of heart-healthy omega-3 fatty acids can be found in the salmon, while quinoa is a complete protein that is high in fibre. In addition to adding a plethora of colours and flavours, the roasted veggies help you meet your recommended daily intake of important vitamins and antioxidants.

Marinate the salmon fillets in a mixture of olive oil, lemon juice, garlic, and fresh herbs such as parsley or dill before grilling to intensify the flavours. For an added flavour boost, you may also mix in some grated Parmesan cheese or coat the roasted vegetables with a balsamic glaze.

Spinach and Strawberry Salad with Grilled Chicken

Ingredients:

- 8 cups baby spinach
- 2 cups fresh strawberries, sliced
- 2 grilled chicken breasts, sliced
- 1/2 cup crumbled feta cheese
- 1/4 cup sliced almonds
- Balsamic vinaigrette dressing

Step-by-Step Preparation Instructions:

1. Preheat your grill or grill pan to medium-high heat and lightly oil the grates.
2. Season the chicken breasts with salt, pepper,

and your desired seasoning blend (such as Italian herbs or lemon pepper).

3. Grill the chicken breasts for about 6-8 minutes per side, or until cooked through and the internal temperature reaches 165°F (74°C). Allow the chicken to rest for 5 minutes before slicing.

4. In a large salad bowl, combine the baby spinach and sliced strawberries.

5. Top the salad with the sliced grilled chicken, crumbled feta cheese, and sliced almonds.

6. Drizzle the desired amount of balsamic vinaigrette dressing over the salad and gently toss to combine.

7. Serve the salad immediately, garnished with additional fresh strawberry slices, if desired.

Nutritional Information (per serving):

- Calories: 320
- Protein: 25g
- Carbohydrates: 18g
- Fiber: 4g
- Fat: 17g

Dietary Recommendation

This vibrant and flavorful salad is an excellent choice for those seeking a light yet satisfying meal. The combination of nutrient-dense spinach, fresh strawberries, lean protein from the grilled chicken, and healthy fats from the feta cheese and almonds creates a well-balanced and delicious dish.

The baby spinach provides a rich source of vitamins A, C, and K, as well as folate and iron. The strawberries not only add a burst of sweetness but also contribute to your daily intake of vitamin C and antioxidants.

Lentil and Sweet Potato Stew

Ingredients:

- 1 cup green lentils, rinsed
- 2 medium sweet potatoes, peeled and diced
- 1 large onion, diced
- 4 cloves garlic, minced
- 4 cups vegetable broth
- 1 (14.5 oz) can diced tomatoes
- 1 teaspoon ground cumin
- 1 teaspoon paprika
- 1/2 teaspoon turmeric
- Salt and freshly ground black pepper, to taste
- Fresh parsley, chopped (for garnish)

Step-by-Step Preparation Instructions:

1. In a large pot or Dutch oven, heat a tablespoon of olive oil over medium heat.

2. Add the diced onion and sauté for 2-3 minutes until translucent.

3. Add the minced garlic and sauté for another minute, until fragrant.

4. Add the rinsed lentils, diced sweet potatoes, vegetable broth, diced tomatoes (with their

juices), cumin, paprika, turmeric, salt, and pepper.

5. Bring the mixture to a boil, then reduce the heat to low, cover, and simmer for 25-30 minutes, or until the lentils and sweet potatoes are tender.

6. If the stew becomes too thick, add a little more vegetable broth or water to reach your desired consistency.

7. Taste and adjust seasoning as needed, adding more salt, pepper, or spices to your liking.

8. Garnish with chopped fresh parsley and serve hot.

Nutritional Information (per serving):

- Calories: 250
- Protein: 12g
- Carbohydrates: 45g
- Fiber: 14g
- Fat: 2g

Dietary Recommendation

This hearty and wholesome lentil and sweet potato stew is a nutritional powerhouse that caters to a variety of dietary preferences, including vegetarian, vegan, and gluten-free diets. It's packed with plant-based protein, fiber, and an array of vitamins and minerals.

The combination of lentils and sweet potatoes provides a satisfying and filling meal, while the blend of spices adds warmth and depth of flavor. The addition of diced tomatoes contributes to the overall nutrient profile, offering vitamin C, lycopene, and a tangy burst of flavor.

Greek Yogurt Parfait with Mixed Berries and Nuts

Ingredients:

- 2 cups Greek yogurt (plain or vanilla)
- 1 cup mixed berries (blueberries, raspberries, strawberries)
- 2 tablespoons honey
- 1/4 cup sliced almonds
- 1/4 cup walnuts, chopped

Step-by-Step Preparation Instructions:

1. In a bowl, combine the mixed berries and honey. Gently toss the berries to coat them evenly with the honey.

2. In a separate bowl or parfait glasses, layer the Greek yogurt, berry mixture, and nuts in an alternating pattern. Start with a layer of yogurt, followed by a layer of berries, then a sprinkle of almonds and walnuts. Repeat the layers until all ingredients are used up.

3. Garnish the top with a few extra berries and a drizzle of honey for added visual appeal.

4. If desired, you can chill the parfaits in the refrigerator for at least 30 minutes before serving to allow the flavors to meld together.

Flavor Enhancer: For an extra burst of flavor, consider

adding a teaspoon of vanilla extract or a pinch of cinnamon to the Greek yogurt before layering.

Nutritional Information (per serving):

- Calories: 250
- Protein: 12g
- Carbohydrates: 26g
- Fiber: 4g
- Fat: 13g
- Saturated Fat: 2g

Dietary Recommendations

This Greek Yogurt Parfait with Mixed Berries and Nuts is an excellent choice for individuals with Myasthenia Gravis. It provides a delightful combination of protein, healthy fats, and carbohydrates, making it a well-balanced and nourishing option.

The Greek yogurt is an excellent source of protein, which is essential for maintaining muscle strength. The mixed berries are rich in antioxidants and fiber, promoting overall health and digestive wellness. The nuts contribute healthy fats and plant-based proteins, further enhancing the nutritional profile of this parfait.

Moreover, this recipe is easy to prepare and can be enjoyed as a satisfying breakfast, snack, or dessert. It is a versatile and convenient option for those with Myasthenia Gravis who may experience difficulty swallowing or chewing.

Baked Cod with Lemon and Herb Sauce

Ingredients:

- 4 cod fillets (6-8 ounces each)
- 1/4 cup fresh lemon juice
- 1/4 cup olive oil
- 4 cloves garlic, minced
- 1/4 cup fresh dill, chopped
- 1/4 cup fresh parsley, chopped
- 1 teaspoon salt
- 1/2 teaspoon black pepper

Step-by-Step Preparation Instructions:

1. Preheat your oven to 400°F (200°C). Line a baking sheet with parchment paper or lightly grease it with cooking spray.

2. In a small bowl, whisk together the lemon juice, olive oil, minced garlic, chopped dill, chopped parsley, salt, and black pepper. Set aside.

3. Place the cod fillets on the prepared baking sheet, ensuring they are spaced apart.

4. Using a pastry brush or a spoon, generously baste the cod fillets with the lemon and herb sauce, making sure to coat them evenly on both sides.

5. Bake the cod in the preheated oven for 12-15 minutes, or until the fish is opaque and flakes easily with a fork.

6. Remove the baked cod from the oven and let it rest for 5 minutes before serving.

7. Drizzle any remaining lemon and herb sauce over the baked cod fillets for added flavor.

Flavor Enhancer: For an extra burst of flavor, you can grate the zest of one lemon and mix it with the lemon and herb sauce before basting the cod.

Nutritional Information (per serving, based on 4 servings):

- Calories: 280
- Protein: 36g
- Carbohydrates: 2g
- Fat: 14g
- Saturated Fat: 2g

Dietary Recommendations

This Baked Cod with Lemon and Herb Sauce is an excellent choice for individuals with Myasthenia Gravis. Cod is a lean and easily digestible protein source, making it a suitable option for those who may experience difficulty swallowing or chewing.

The lemon and herb sauce adds a burst of flavor while providing additional nutritional benefits. Lemon is rich in vitamin C, which supports a healthy immune system, while the fresh herbs contribute valuable antioxidants and phytochemicals.

This dish is also low in saturated fat and cholesterol,

aligning with the dietary recommendations for Myasthenia Gravis patients. The olive oil used in the sauce provides healthy monounsaturated fats, which can help maintain overall health.

Vegetable and Tofu Stir-Fry with Brown Rice

Ingredients:

- 1 block (14 ounces) extra-firm tofu, drained and cut into 1-inch cubes
- 2 cups broccoli florets
- 1 red bell pepper, sliced
- 1 cup sliced carrots
- 2 cloves garlic, minced
- 1 tablespoon grated fresh ginger
- 2 tablespoons low-sodium soy sauce
- 1 tablespoon sesame oil
- 2 cups cooked brown rice

Step-by-Step Preparation Instructions:

1. Press the tofu cubes between paper towels or a clean kitchen towel to remove excess moisture.

2. In a large skillet or wok, heat 1 tablespoon of sesame oil over medium-high heat.

3. Add the tofu cubes and stir-fry for 5-7 minutes, or until lightly browned on all sides. Remove the tofu from the skillet and set it aside.

4. In the same skillet, add the remaining 1 tablespoon of sesame oil and heat it over medium-high heat.

5. Add the minced garlic and grated ginger, and stir-fry for 30 seconds, or until fragrant.

6. Add the broccoli florets, sliced bell pepper, and sliced carrots to the skillet. Stir-fry for 5-7 minutes, or until the vegetables are tender-crisp.

7. Return the tofu cubes to the skillet and add the low-sodium soy sauce. Toss everything together to combine and ensure the tofu and vegetables are evenly coated with the sauce.

8. Serve the vegetable and tofu stir-fry hot, over a bed of cooked brown rice.

Flavor Enhancer: For an extra kick of flavor, consider adding a teaspoon of red pepper flakes or a drizzle of toasted sesame oil to the stir-fry.

Nutritional Information (per serving, based on 4 servings):

- Calories: 310
- Protein: 16g
- Carbohydrates: 38g
- Fiber: 6g
- Fat: 12g

- Saturated Fat: 1g

Dietary Recommendations

This Vegetable and Tofu Stir-Fry with Brown Rice is an excellent choice for individuals with Myasthenia Gravis. It is a well-balanced dish that provides a variety of nutrients while being easy to chew and swallow.

Tofu is an excellent source of plant-based protein, which is essential for maintaining muscle strength. The combination of vegetables, such as broccoli, bell peppers, and carrots, provides a rich array of vitamins, minerals, and antioxidants.

Grilled Chicken Salad with Avocado and Balsamic Vinaigrette

Ingredients:

- 4 boneless, skinless chicken breasts
- Salt and black pepper, to taste
- 8 cups mixed greens
- 2 cups cherry tomatoes, halved
- 2 ripe avocados, pitted and sliced
- 1/4 cup balsamic vinegar
- 2 tablespoons olive oil

- 1 tablespoon Dijon mustard
- 1 tablespoon honey

Step-by-Step Preparation Instructions:

1. Preheat your grill to medium-high heat or preheat your oven to 400°F (200°C) if using an oven grill pan.

2. Season the chicken breasts with salt and black pepper on both sides.

3. Grill the chicken breasts for about 6-8 minutes per side, or until cooked through and the internal temperature reaches 165°F (74°C). Let the chicken rest for 5 minutes before slicing.

4. In a small bowl, whisk together the balsamic vinegar, olive oil, Dijon mustard, and honey to create the vinaigrette dressing.

5. In a large salad bowl, combine the mixed greens, cherry tomatoes, sliced avocado, and grilled chicken strips.

6. Drizzle the balsamic vinaigrette over the salad and gently toss to coat.

Flavour Enhancer (Optional): Add a sprinkle of fresh herbs like basil or parsley for an extra burst of flavor.

Nutritional Information (per serving):

- Calories: 420
- Total Fat: 22g
- Saturated Fat: 4g
- Cholesterol: 85mg

- Sodium: 220mg
- Total Carbohydrates: 24g
- Dietary Fiber: 9g
- Protein: 34g

Dietary Recommendation

This salad is an excellent choice for those following a balanced diet. It provides lean protein from the grilled chicken, healthy fats from the avocado and olive oil, and a variety of vitamins and minerals from the mixed greens and cherry tomatoes. The balsamic vinaigrette adds a tangy and slightly sweet flavor profile without excessive amounts of sugar or unhealthy fats.

Grilling the chicken breast not only adds a delicious smoky flavor but also keeps the preparation method lean and healthy. For those with swallowing difficulties, the chicken can be sliced or diced into smaller pieces to make it easier to consume.

This salad can be enjoyed as a main course or a substantial side dish, making it a versatile and satisfying option for any meal. Adjust the portion sizes as needed to suit your individual dietary requirements.

Quinoa and Black Bean Salad

Ingredients:

- 1 cup uncooked quinoa
- 1 (15 oz) can black beans, rinsed and drained
- 1 cup frozen corn kernels, thawed

- 1 red bell pepper, diced
- 1/2 red onion, diced
- 1/4 cup chopped fresh cilantro
- 3 tablespoons lime juice
- 2 tablespoons olive oil
- Salt and black pepper, to taste

Step-by-Step Preparation Instructions:

1. Cook the quinoa according to package instructions. Once cooked, fluff with a fork and let it cool completely.

2. In a large mixing bowl, combine the cooked and cooled quinoa, black beans, corn, diced bell pepper, diced red onion, and chopped cilantro.

3. In a small bowl, whisk together the lime juice, olive oil, salt, and black pepper to create the dressing.

4. Pour the dressing over the quinoa mixture and gently toss to coat all the ingredients evenly.

Flavour Enhancer (Optional): Add a sprinkle of cumin or chili powder for an extra kick of flavor.

Nutritional Information (per serving):

- Calories: 210
- Total Fat: 6g
- Saturated Fat: 1g
- Cholesterol: 0mg
- Sodium: 120mg

- Total Carbohydrates: 33g
- Dietary Fiber: 8g
- Protein: 8g

Dietary Recommendation

This quinoa and black bean salad is a nutrient-dense and filling dish that's perfect for those following a plant-based or vegetarian diet. It's rich in fiber, protein, and various vitamins and minerals, making it a well-balanced meal option.

Quinoa is a gluten-free grain that provides a good source of plant-based protein, while black beans offer additional protein, fiber, and essential nutrients like iron and folate. The combination of fresh vegetables and herbs adds a burst of flavors and textures, making this salad both delicious and satisfying.

For those with swallowing difficulties, the ingredients in this salad can be easily modified. The quinoa and black beans can be mashed or pureed, while the vegetables can be finely chopped or blended into the dressing.

This salad can be served as a main dish or a side, and it's perfect for meal prepping as the flavors will continue to develop and intensify over time. Consider adding grilled chicken or fish for an extra protein boost, or enjoy it as a refreshing vegetarian option.

Baked Sweet Potato with Spinach and Feta

Ingredients:

- 4 medium sweet potatoes
- 2 cups fresh baby spinach
- 1/2 cup crumbled feta cheese
- 2 tablespoons olive oil
- 2 cloves garlic, minced
- Salt and black pepper, to taste

Step-by-Step Preparation Instructions:

1. Preheat your oven to 400°F (200°C).

2. Scrub the sweet potatoes and prick them several times with a fork. Place them on a baking sheet lined with parchment paper or foil.

3. Bake the sweet potatoes for 45-60 minutes, or until they are tender when pierced with a fork.

4. While the sweet potatoes are baking, heat the olive oil in a skillet over medium heat. Add the minced garlic and sauté for 1 minute until fragrant.

5. Add the fresh baby spinach to the skillet and cook for 2-3 minutes, or until the spinach is wilted. Season with salt and black pepper to taste.

6. Once the sweet potatoes are cooked, remove them from the oven and let them cool slightly. Cut each sweet potato in half lengthwise and create a well in the center.

7. Spoon the sautéed spinach mixture into the wells of the sweet potatoes, dividing it evenly among the halves.

8. Top each sweet potato half with crumbled feta cheese.

Flavour Enhancer (Optional): Sprinkle with a pinch of nutmeg or paprika for an extra burst of flavor.

Nutritional Information (per serving):

- Calories: 280
- Total Fat: 10g
- Saturated Fat: 3g
- Cholesterol: 15mg
- Sodium: 320mg
- Total Carbohydrates: 42g
- Dietary Fiber: 6g
- Protein: 7g

Dietary Recommendation

This baked sweet potato with spinach and feta dish is a delightful combination of flavors and textures. Sweet potatoes are an excellent source of complex carbohydrates, fiber, and various vitamins and minerals, including beta-carotene and vitamin C.

The addition of fresh baby spinach provides a nutrient-dense boost of vitamins, minerals, and antioxidants, while the feta cheese adds a tangy and creamy element, as well as a source of protein and calcium.

For those with swallowing difficulties, the ingredients in

this dish can be easily modified. The sweet potatoes can be mashed or pureed, while the spinach and feta can be finely chopped or blended into the sweet potato mixture.

This dish can be served as a main course or a side, and it's versatile enough to be enjoyed for breakfast, lunch, or dinner. Consider adding grilled chicken or fish for an extra protein boost, or enjoy it as a satisfying vegetarian option.

Zucchini Noodles with Tomato and Basil

Ingredients:

- 4 medium zucchini, spiralized or julienned into noodles
- 2 cups cherry tomatoes, halved
- 1/2 cup fresh basil leaves, chopped
- 4 garlic cloves, minced
- 1/4 cup olive oil
- 2 tablespoons balsamic vinegar
- Salt and freshly ground black pepper, to taste

Step-by-Step Preparation Instructions:

1. In a large bowl, combine the zucchini noodles, cherry tomatoes, chopped basil, and minced garlic.
2. In a small bowl, whisk together the olive oil and balsamic vinegar. Season with salt and pepper to taste.

3. Pour the vinaigrette over the zucchini noodle mixture and toss gently to combine, ensuring all the ingredients are evenly coated.

4. Let the salad sit for 5-10 minutes to allow the flavors to meld together.

5. Taste and adjust seasoning if needed, adding more salt, pepper, or a splash of balsamic vinegar to your liking.

6. **Flavor Enhancer (Optional):** For an extra burst of flavor, you can grate a tablespoon or two of Parmesan cheese over the salad before serving.

Nutritional Information (Per Serving):

- Calories: 220
- Total Fat: 18g
- Saturated Fat: 2.5g
- Cholesterol: 0mg
- Sodium: 120mg
- Total Carbohydrates: 13g
- Dietary Fiber: 3g
- Sugars: 7g
- Protein: 4g

Dietary Recommendation

This refreshing and light zucchini noodle salad is an excellent choice for those following a low-carb or gluten-free diet. It's also an ideal dish for individuals with myasthenia gravis, as it's easy to chew and swallow, and the zucchini noodles provide a good source of potassium, which is essential for proper muscle function.

The addition of fresh basil and cherry tomatoes not only adds flavor but also provides a boost of vitamins and antioxidants, while the olive oil and balsamic vinegar dressing offers a healthy dose of monounsaturated fats.

Grilled Chicken and Vegetable Skewers

Ingredients:

- 1 lb boneless, skinless chicken breasts, cut into 1-inch cubes
- 2 bell peppers (mix of colors), cut into 1-inch pieces
- 2 medium zucchini, sliced into 1/2-inch rounds
- 1 red onion, cut into wedges
- 1/4 cup olive oil
- 2 tablespoons fresh lemon juice
- 2 cloves garlic, minced
- 1 teaspoon dried thyme
- 1 teaspoon dried rosemary
- Salt and freshly ground black pepper, to taste

Step-by-Step Preparation Instructions:

1. In a large bowl, combine the cubed chicken, bell pepper pieces, zucchini rounds, and red onion wedges.
2. In a small bowl, whisk together the olive oil,

lemon juice, minced garlic, dried thyme, dried rosemary, salt, and black pepper to create the marinade.

3. Pour the marinade over the chicken and vegetable mixture, tossing gently to coat evenly. Cover and refrigerate for at least 30 minutes, or up to 2 hours, to allow the flavors to meld.

4. Preheat your grill or grill pan to medium-high heat.

5. Thread the marinated chicken and vegetables onto skewers, alternating between chicken, bell peppers, zucchini, and red onion.

6. Grill the skewers for about 12-15 minutes, turning occasionally, until the chicken is cooked through and the vegetables are tender and lightly charred.

7. **Flavor Enhancer (Optional):** Squeeze fresh lemon juice over the skewers before serving for an extra burst of citrusy flavor.

Nutritional Information (Per Skewer):

- Calories: 280
- Total Fat: 14g
- Saturated Fat: 2g
- Cholesterol: 65mg
- Sodium: 120mg
- Total Carbohydrates: 12g
- Dietary Fiber: 3g
- Sugars: 6g
- Protein: 26g

Dietary Recommendation

These grilled chicken and vegetable skewers are an excellent choice for those following a myasthenia gravis diet. The lean protein from the chicken and the nutrient-dense vegetables make for a well-balanced and satisfying meal. The marinade adds flavor without relying on excessive amounts of salt or sugar.

The zucchini and bell peppers provide a good source of potassium, which is essential for muscle function, while the lemon juice and olive oil in the marinade offer a healthy dose of vitamin C and monounsaturated fats, respectively.

Tuna and White Bean Salad

Ingredients:

- 2 (5 oz) cans tuna, drained
- 1 (15 oz) can white beans, drained and rinsed
- 1 cup cherry tomatoes, halved
- 1/2 red onion, thinly sliced
- 1/4 cup fresh parsley, chopped
- 3 tablespoons lemon juice
- 2 tablespoons olive oil
- Salt and freshly ground black pepper, to taste

Step-by-Step Preparation Instructions:

1. In a large bowl, gently flake the drained tuna with a fork, breaking it into smaller pieces.
2. Add the drained and rinsed white beans,

halved cherry tomatoes, thinly sliced red onion, and chopped parsley to the bowl.

3. In a small bowl, whisk together the lemon juice and olive oil. Season with salt and pepper to taste.

4. Pour the lemon-olive oil dressing over the tuna and white bean mixture, and gently toss to combine, ensuring all the ingredients are evenly coated.

5. Let the salad sit for 10-15 minutes to allow the flavors to meld together.

6. Taste and adjust seasoning if needed, adding more lemon juice, salt, or pepper to your liking.

7. **Flavor Enhancer (Optional):** For an extra kick of flavor, you can add a tablespoon or two of finely chopped fresh herbs like dill, chives, or basil.

Nutritional Information (Per Serving):

- Calories: 270
- Total Fat: 8g
- Saturated Fat: 1g
- Cholesterol: 30mg
- Sodium: 350mg
- Total Carbohydrates: 25g
- Dietary Fiber: 7g
- Sugars: 3g
- Protein: 25g

Dietary Recommendation

This tuna and white bean salad is a nutrient-dense and satisfying meal that is perfect for those following a myasthenia gravis diet. The combination of lean protein from the tuna and the fiber-rich white beans makes for a filling and well-balanced dish.

The addition of fresh parsley, cherry tomatoes, and red onion not only adds flavor but also provides a boost of vitamins, antioxidants, and potassium, which is essential for proper muscle function.

Avocado and Egg Toast

Ingredients:

- 4 slices of whole-grain bread
- 2 ripe avocados
- 4 large eggs
- Salt and freshly ground black pepper, to taste
- 1 tablespoon extra-virgin olive oil (optional)
- 1 teaspoon fresh lemon juice (optional)
- Chopped fresh herbs like parsley, chives, or dill (optional)

Step-by-Step Preparation Instructions:

1. Toast the whole-grain bread slices until golden brown and crispy.

2. Halve the avocados, remove the pits, and scoop the flesh into a bowl. Mash the avocado

with a fork until it reaches a slightly chunky consistency.

3. If desired, season the mashed avocado with a drizzle of olive oil, a squeeze of fresh lemon juice, and a pinch of salt and pepper. Mix well to combine.

4. In a non-stick skillet or pan, crack the eggs and cook them over low to medium heat, using your preferred cooking method (such as sunny-side up, over-easy, or scrambled).

5. Spread the mashed avocado evenly over the toasted bread slices.

6. Top each avocado toast with a cooked egg.

7. Season with additional salt and pepper, if desired, and garnish with chopped fresh herbs of your choice.

Nutritional Information (per serving):

- Calories: 320
- Total Fat: 18g
- Saturated Fat: 3g
- Cholesterol: 185mg
- Sodium: 280mg
- Total Carbohydrates: 28g
- Dietary Fiber: 7g
- Protein: 12g

Dietary Recommendation

This avocado and egg toast recipe is a perfect combination of healthy fats, protein, and complex carbohydrates, making it a nutritious and satisfying meal option. The whole-grain bread provides fiber and sustained energy, while the avocado offers heart-healthy monounsaturated fats and essential nutrients. The eggs are an excellent source of protein, which can help promote feelings of fullness and support muscle maintenance.

To enhance the flavor and nutrition profile, you can experiment with different seasoning options or add fresh herbs like parsley, chives, or dill. Additionally, consider incorporating a drizzle of olive oil or a squeeze of lemon juice to add depth and brightness to the flavors.

For individuals with myasthenia gravis, this recipe can be easily adjusted to meet specific dietary needs. The avocado and egg can be mashed together for easier swallowing, or the toast can be moistened with a bit of olive oil or avocado mash to soften the texture. Remember to consult with your healthcare provider for personalized dietary recommendations based on your condition and individual needs.

Grilled Salmon and Asparagus Salad

Ingredients:

- 4 (6-ounce) salmon fillets
- 1 bunch of fresh asparagus, trimmed

- 6 cups mixed greens (such as arugula, spinach, and romaine lettuce)
- 1 cup cherry tomatoes, halved
- 1 English cucumber, sliced
- 1/4 cup balsamic vinaigrette dressing (or your preferred vinaigrette)
- Salt and freshly ground black pepper, to taste
- Olive oil or cooking spray for grilling

Step-by-Step Preparation Instructions:

1. Preheat an outdoor grill or indoor grill pan to medium-high heat. Brush or spray the grill grates with olive oil or cooking spray.

2. Season the salmon fillets with salt and pepper on both sides.

3. Grill the salmon fillets for about 4-6 minutes per side, or until they reach the desired doneness.

4. While the salmon is grilling, toss the asparagus with a drizzle of olive oil and season with salt and pepper.

5. Place the asparagus spears on the grill and cook for 3-5 minutes, turning occasionally, until they are tender and slightly charred.

6. Remove the grilled salmon and asparagus from the grill and set them aside to cool slightly.

7. In a large salad bowl, combine the mixed greens, cherry tomatoes, and sliced cucumber.

8. Drizzle the balsamic vinaigrette dressing over

the salad and toss gently to coat.

9. Arrange the grilled salmon fillets and asparagus spears over the salad.

10. Serve immediately and enjoy!

Nutritional Information (per serving):

- Calories: 420
- Total Fat: 20g
- Saturated Fat: 3g
- Cholesterol: 90mg
- Sodium: 280mg
- Total Carbohydrates: 16g
- Dietary Fiber: 5g
- Protein: 40g

Dietary Recommendation

This grilled salmon and asparagus salad is a delightful and nutritious meal that combines lean protein, fiber-rich vegetables, and heart-healthy fats. The salmon is an excellent source of omega-3 fatty acids, which have anti-inflammatory properties and may benefit individuals with myasthenia gravis. The asparagus is a nutrient-dense vegetable that provides fiber, folate, and antioxidants.

To make this dish more accessible for individuals with swallowing difficulties, the salmon can be flaked or shredded, and the asparagus can be cut into smaller pieces or pureed. Additionally, the dressing can be drizzled over the entire salad to moisten the ingredients and make them easier to swallow.

For those looking to increase their potassium intake, consider adding sliced avocado or roasted sweet potatoes to the salad. These nutrient-rich ingredients can help replenish potassium levels, which may be beneficial for individuals with myasthenia gravis.

Remember to consult with your healthcare provider for personalized dietary recommendations based on your specific condition and individual needs.

Quinoa and Roasted Vegetable Bowl

Ingredients:

- 1 cup uncooked quinoa
- 2 cups broccoli florets
- 2 cups cauliflower florets
- 2 bell peppers (any color), sliced
- 4 cloves garlic, minced
- 3 tablespoons olive oil
- 2 tablespoons fresh lemon juice
- Salt and freshly ground black pepper, to taste
- Chopped fresh parsley or cilantro for garnish (optional)

Step-by-Step Preparation Instructions:

1. Preheat your oven to 400°F (200°C).
2. Rinse the quinoa under cold water and drain

it well. Transfer the rinsed quinoa to a saucepan, add 2 cups of water, and bring it to a boil. Reduce the heat to low, cover, and simmer for 15-20 minutes, or until all the water is absorbed and the quinoa is fluffy.

3. On a large baking sheet, spread out the broccoli florets, cauliflower florets, and sliced bell peppers. Drizzle with 2 tablespoons of olive oil and sprinkle with minced garlic, salt, and pepper. Toss to coat the vegetables evenly.

4. Roast the vegetables in the preheated oven for 20-25 minutes, or until they are tender and slightly charred, stirring occasionally.

5. Once the quinoa is cooked, fluff it with a fork and transfer it to a large serving bowl.

6. Add the roasted vegetables to the quinoa and drizzle with the remaining 1 tablespoon of olive oil and fresh lemon juice. Toss gently to combine.

7. Garnish with chopped fresh parsley or cilantro, if desired.

8. Serve warm or at room temperature and enjoy!

Nutritional Information (per serving):

- Calories: 330
- Total Fat: 14g
- Saturated Fat: 2g
- Cholesterol: 0mg
- Sodium: 120mg
- Total Carbohydrates: 45g

- Dietary Fiber: 8g
- Protein: 10g

Lentil and Vegetable Soup

Ingredients:

- 1 cup dried lentils (green or brown)
- 4 large carrots, peeled and diced
- 3 celery stalks, diced
- 1 large onion, diced
- 4 cloves garlic, minced
- 6 cups vegetable broth
- 1 (14.5 oz) can diced tomatoes
- 1 bay leaf
- 1 teaspoon dried thyme
- Salt and freshly ground black pepper, to taste
- 2 tablespoons fresh parsley, chopped (for garnish)

Step-by-Step Preparation Instructions:

1. Rinse the lentils under cold water and pick out any debris or shriveled lentils.

2. In a large pot or Dutch oven, combine the lentils, carrots, celery, onion, garlic, vegetable broth, diced tomatoes, bay leaf, and thyme. Season with salt and pepper to taste.

3. Bring the mixture to a boil over high heat,

then reduce the heat to low, cover, and simmer for 25-30 minutes, or until the lentils and vegetables are tender.

4. Remove the bay leaf and discard it. If the soup is too thick, add a little more vegetable broth or water to reach your desired consistency.

5. Taste and adjust seasoning with salt and pepper as needed.

6. Ladle the soup into bowls and garnish with chopped fresh parsley.

Flavor Enhancer: For an extra depth of flavor, you can sauté the onions and garlic in a tablespoon of olive oil before adding the other ingredients. This will bring out their natural sweetness and aroma.

Nutritional Information (per serving, based on 6 servings):

- Calories: 180
- Total Fat: 1g
- Saturated Fat: 0g
- Cholesterol: 0mg
- Sodium: 480mg
- Total Carbohydrates: 32g
- Dietary Fiber: 12g
- Protein: 11g

Dietary Recommendation

This lentil and vegetable soup is a nutrient-dense and fiber-rich meal that aligns perfectly with the dietary guidelines for those living with Myasthenia

Gravis. Lentils are an excellent source of plant-based protein and are easy to digest, making them an ideal choice for individuals with swallowing difficulties. The combination of vegetables provides a variety of vitamins, minerals, and antioxidants, while the vegetable broth adds flavor without the need for excessive salt. This soup can be easily thickened or thinned to suit individual preferences, ensuring a comfortable and safe eating experience. Enjoy this comforting and nourishing soup as a satisfying main course or as a side dish to complement other meals. Remember to stay hydrated and consult with your healthcare provider for personalized dietary recommendations.

Baked Chicken with Roasted Potatoes and Brussels Sprouts

Ingredients:

- 4 boneless, skinless chicken breasts
- 1 pound small red potatoes, quartered
- 1 pound Brussels sprouts, trimmed and halved
- 4 tablespoons olive oil, divided
- 3 cloves garlic, minced
- 2 teaspoons dried rosemary
- 1 teaspoon dried thyme
- Salt and freshly ground black pepper, to taste

Step-by-Step Preparation Instructions:

1. Preheat your oven to 400°F (200°C).

2. In a large bowl, toss the quartered potatoes with 2 tablespoons of olive oil, half of the minced garlic, 1 teaspoon of dried rosemary, and a pinch of salt and pepper. Spread the potatoes onto a baking sheet in a single layer.

3. In the same bowl, toss the halved Brussels sprouts with the remaining 2 tablespoons of olive oil, the remaining minced garlic, 1 teaspoon of dried rosemary, 1 teaspoon of dried thyme, and salt and pepper to taste. Spread the Brussels sprouts onto a separate baking sheet in a single layer.

4. Place the chicken breasts in a baking dish and season them with salt, pepper, and the remaining dried thyme.

5. Roast the potatoes and Brussels sprouts in the preheated oven for 15 minutes.

6. After 15 minutes, remove the baking sheets from the oven and carefully toss the vegetables to promote even browning.

7. Place the baking dish with the seasoned chicken breasts in the oven alongside the vegetables and continue roasting for an additional 20-25 minutes, or until the chicken reaches an internal temperature of 165°F (74°C) and the vegetables are tender and lightly caramelized.

8. Remove everything from the oven and allow

the chicken to rest for 5 minutes before serving.

9. Arrange the roasted potatoes and Brussels sprouts on a platter, and place the baked chicken breasts on top or alongside them.

Flavor Enhancer: For an extra burst of flavor, you can squeeze fresh lemon juice over the roasted vegetables and chicken just before serving.

Nutritional Information (per serving, based on 4 servings):

- Calories: 420
- Total Fat: 18g
- Saturated Fat: 3g
- Cholesterol: 100mg
- Sodium: 180mg
- Total Carbohydrates: 30g
- Dietary Fiber: 6g
- Protein: 36g

Dietary Recommendation

This baked chicken dish with roasted potatoes and Brussels sprouts is a well-balanced and nutrient-dense meal that adheres to the dietary guidelines for individuals with Myasthenia Gravis. The lean protein from the chicken provides essential amino acids for muscle maintenance, while the potatoes and Brussels sprouts offer a good source of complex carbohydrates, fiber, and various vitamins and minerals. The use of olive oil and herbs adds flavor without excessive salt or saturated fats. This dish can be easily modified by adjusting the portion sizes or substituting ingredients to suit individual preferences and dietary needs. Enjoy this wholesome and satisfying meal as a complete dinner or as a versatile component of a varied diet plan. Remember to stay hydrated and consult with your healthcare provider for personalized dietary recommendations.

Greek Salad with Grilled Shrimp

Ingredients:

- 1 pound large shrimp, peeled and deveined
- 2 tablespoons olive oil, plus extra for brushing
- 1 teaspoon dried oregano
- Salt and freshly ground black pepper, to taste
- 1 head romaine lettuce, chopped
- 1 pint cherry tomatoes, halved
- 1 English cucumber, diced
- 1/2 red onion, thinly sliced
- 1/2 cup crumbled feta cheese
- 1/2 cup Kalamata olives, pitted and halved
- 1/4 cup Greek dressing (or vinaigrette of your

choice)

Step-by-Step Preparation Instructions:

1. Preheat an outdoor grill or indoor grill pan to medium-high heat.

2. In a bowl, toss the shrimp with 2 tablespoons of olive oil, dried oregano, salt, and pepper until well coated.

3. Brush the grill grates with a little olive oil to prevent sticking.

4. Grill the shrimp for 2-3 minutes per side, or until they turn opaque and slightly charred. Remove from heat and set aside to cool slightly.

5. In a large salad bowl, combine the chopped romaine lettuce, cherry tomatoes, diced cucumber, sliced red onion, crumbled feta cheese, and Kalamata olives.

6. Drizzle the Greek dressing (or vinaigrette of your choice) over the salad and toss gently to coat evenly.

7. Arrange the grilled shrimp on top of the salad or serve them alongside.

Flavor Enhancer: For an extra burst of flavor, you can add a squeeze of fresh lemon juice over the salad and shrimp just before serving.

Nutritional Information (per serving, based on 4 servings):

- Calories: 320
- Total Fat: 18g

- Saturated Fat: 4g
- Cholesterol: 180mg
- Sodium: 880mg
- Total Carbohydrates:

Quinoa and Roasted Vegetable Stuffed Bell Peppers

Ingredients:

- 4 large bell peppers (any color)
- 1 cup cooked quinoa
- 1 small zucchini, diced and roasted
- 1 small eggplant, diced and roasted
- 1 cup diced tomatoes
- 3 cloves garlic, minced
- 2 tablespoons fresh basil, chopped
- 2 tablespoons fresh parsley, chopped
- 1/4 cup grated Parmesan cheese
- Salt and pepper to taste
- 2 tablespoons olive oil

Step-by-Step Preparation Instructions:

1. Preheat your oven to 375°F (190°C).

2. Cut the tops off the bell peppers and remove the seeds and membranes. Place the peppers in a baking dish and set aside.

3. In a large bowl, combine the cooked quinoa, roasted zucchini, roasted eggplant,

diced tomatoes, minced garlic, chopped basil, chopped parsley, and grated Parmesan cheese. Season with salt and pepper to taste.

4. Drizzle the olive oil over the bell peppers, both inside and out, and rub it evenly over the peppers.

5. Stuff the bell peppers with the quinoa and vegetable mixture, packing it down gently.

6. Cover the baking dish with aluminum foil and bake for 30 minutes.

7. Remove the foil and bake for an additional 15-20 minutes, or until the peppers are tender and the filling is heated through.

Flavor Enhancer: For an extra flavor boost, you can add a drizzle of balsamic glaze or a sprinkle of red pepper flakes over the stuffed peppers before serving.

Nutritional Information (per serving):

- Calories: 250
- Total Fat: 10g
- Saturated Fat: 2g
- Cholesterol: 5mg
- Sodium: 200mg
- Total Carbohydrates: 35g
- Dietary Fiber: 8g
- Protein: 8g

Dietary Recommendation

These quinoa and roasted vegetable stuffed bell peppers are a nutritious and flavorful meal that aligns with the recommended dietary guidelines. They are low in fat and cholesterol, while providing a good source of fiber, protein, and an array of vitamins and minerals from the vegetables.

This dish is perfect for those following a plant-based diet or looking to incorporate more meatless meals into their routine. The quinoa provides a satisfying protein boost, while the roasted vegetables add depth of flavor and a pleasing texture.

Grilled Portobello Mushroom Caps with Spinach and Feta

Ingredients:

- 4 large portobello mushroom caps, stems removed
- 1 cup fresh spinach leaves, washed and stems removed
- 1/2 cup crumbled feta cheese
- 3 cloves garlic, minced
- 2 tablespoons balsamic vinegar
- 2 tablespoons olive oil
- Salt and freshly ground black pepper, to taste

Step-by-Step Preparation Instructions:

1. Preheat your grill or grill pan to medium-high

heat.

2. Brush the portobello mushroom caps with olive oil on both sides and season with salt and pepper.

3. Grill the mushroom caps for about 4-5 minutes per side, or until they are tender and grill marks appear.

4. In a small bowl, mix together the spinach leaves, feta cheese, minced garlic, and balsamic vinegar. Season with salt and pepper to taste.

5. Once the mushroom caps are grilled, remove them from the heat and place them on a serving plate.

6. Evenly distribute the spinach-feta mixture on top of each mushroom cap.

7. Serve hot and enjoy!

Flavour Enhancer (Optional): Sprinkle a pinch of red pepper flakes or drizzle with a bit of lemon juice for an added kick of flavor.

Nutritional Information (per serving):

- Calories: 210
- Total Fat: 14g
- Saturated Fat: 4g
- Cholesterol: 20mg
- Sodium: 420mg
- Total Carbohydrates: 14g
- Dietary Fiber: 4g
- Protein: 9g

Dietary Recommendation

This grilled portobello mushroom dish is a delightful vegetarian option that aligns perfectly with the dietary guidelines for Americans. It is low in saturated fat and cholesterol, while offering a good source of fiber and protein from the mushrooms, spinach, and feta cheese.

The combination of flavors from the balsamic vinegar, garlic, and feta creates a delightful Mediterranean flair, making this dish both nutritious and satisfying. It can be served as a main course or as a side dish, making it a versatile addition to any meal.

Vegetable and Lentil Curry

Ingredients:

- 1 cup red lentils, rinsed
- 1 can (14.5 oz) diced tomatoes
- 1 can (13.5 oz) coconut milk
- 1 large onion, diced
- 4 cloves garlic, minced
- 1 tablespoon fresh grated ginger
- 2 tablespoons curry powder
- 1 teaspoon ground cumin
- 1 teaspoon ground coriander
- 1/2 teaspoon cayenne pepper (optional, for

heat)

- 2 cups vegetable broth or water
- 2 carrots, peeled and sliced
- 1 bell pepper, diced
- 2 cups fresh spinach or kale, roughly chopped
- Salt and black pepper, to taste
- Fresh cilantro or parsley for garnish (optional)

Step-by-Step Preparation Instructions:

1. Rinse the lentils under cold water and set aside.

2. In a large pot or Dutch oven, heat a tablespoon of olive oil over medium heat. Add the diced onion and sauté for 2-3 minutes until translucent.

3. Add the minced garlic and grated ginger to the pot, and cook for another minute, stirring frequently to prevent burning.

4. Stir in the curry powder, cumin, coriander, and cayenne pepper (if using), and cook for 30 seconds to toast the spices.

5. Pour in the diced tomatoes (with their juices), coconut milk, and vegetable broth or water. Add the rinsed lentils and sliced carrots.

6. Bring the mixture to a boil, then reduce the heat to low, cover, and simmer for 20 minutes, stirring occasionally.

7. After 20 minutes, stir in the diced bell pepper

and spinach or kale. Continue simmering for 5-10 minutes, or until the lentils and vegetables are tender.

8. Taste and adjust seasoning with salt and black pepper as needed.

9. Garnish with fresh cilantro or parsley (if desired) and serve hot over basmati rice or with naan bread.

Flavor Enhancer (Optional): For an extra burst of flavor, you can add 1-2 tablespoons of freshly grated lemon or lime zest to the curry.

Nutritional Information (per serving):

- Calories: 280
- Protein: 12g
- Carbohydrates: 40g
- Fiber: 14g
- Fat: 10g

Dietary Recommendation

This vegetable and lentil curry is a nutritious, plant-based dish that is rich in fiber, protein, and essential vitamins and minerals. It's a great choice for those following a vegetarian or vegan diet, as well as for anyone looking to incorporate more meatless meals into their routine.

The combination of lentils, vegetables, and coconut milk provides a satisfying and well-balanced meal that is low in saturated fat and cholesterol. The addition of curry powder and other aromatic spices adds depth of flavor and can help to boost metabolism.

For those with myasthenia gravis or swallowing difficulties, the lentils and vegetables can be easily pureed or mashed to create a smoother consistency. You can also adjust the spice level to suit your preferences by reducing or omitting the cayenne pepper.

Baked Salmon with Pesto and Roasted Potatoes

Ingredients:

For the Salmon:

- 4 (6-ounce) salmon fillets, skin-on
- 1/4 cup pesto sauce (homemade or store-bought)
- 1 tablespoon olive oil
- Salt and freshly ground black pepper, to taste

For the Roasted Potatoes:

- 1 pound small potatoes (such as Yukon Gold or red potatoes), quartered
- 2 tablespoons olive oil
- 1 teaspoon dried rosemary
- 1 teaspoon dried thyme
- Salt and freshly ground black pepper, to taste

Step-by-Step Preparation Instructions:

1. Preheat your oven to 400°F (200°C).
2. Prepare the Roasted Potatoes:

- In a large bowl, toss the quartered potatoes with 2 tablespoons of olive oil, dried rosemary, dried thyme, salt, and pepper until well-coated.
- Spread the potatoes in a single layer on a baking sheet lined with parchment paper or a silicone baking mat.
- Roast in the preheated oven for 25-30 minutes, or until the potatoes are golden brown and tender, stirring halfway through the cooking time.

3. Prepare the Salmon:

- Rinse the salmon fillets under cold water and pat them dry with paper towels.
- Place the salmon fillets, skin-side down, on a parchment-lined baking sheet or a greased baking dish.
- Brush the top of each fillet with olive oil and season with salt and pepper.
- Spread the pesto sauce evenly over the top of each salmon fillet.

4. Bake the Salmon:

- Once the potatoes have been roasting for 15 minutes, place the baking sheet or dish with the prepared salmon fillets on the middle rack of the oven.

- Bake the salmon for 12-15 minutes, or until it flakes easily with a fork and reaches an internal temperature of 145°F (63°C).

5. Flavour Enhancer (Optional):

- For an extra burst of flavor, you can squeeze fresh lemon juice over the baked salmon fillets just before serving.

Nutritional Information (per serving):

- Calories: 470
- Total Fat: 24g
- Saturated Fat: 4g
- Cholesterol: 85mg
- Sodium: 380mg
- Total Carbohydrates: 28g
- Dietary Fiber: 3g
- Protein: 34g

Dietary Recommendation

This baked salmon with pesto and roasted potatoes is a nutritious and delicious meal that aligns with the dietary guidelines for Myasthenia Gravis patients. The salmon provides lean protein, while the pesto sauce adds a flavorful punch of healthy fats from olive oil and nuts. The roasted potatoes offer a comforting source of complex carbohydrates and fiber.

For Myasthenia Gravis patients, this meal is easy to chew and swallow, thanks to the tender baked salmon and soft roasted potatoes. The potatoes can be easily mashed or cut into smaller pieces if needed.

Mediterranean Chickpea Salad

Ingredients:

- 1 (15 oz) can chickpeas, drained and rinsed
- 1 cup cherry tomatoes, halved
- 1 small cucumber, diced
- 1/2 red onion, thinly sliced
- 1/2 cup crumbled feta cheese
- 1/4 cup chopped fresh parsley
- 3 tablespoons fresh lemon juice
- 2 tablespoons extra-virgin olive oil
- 1/4 teaspoon salt
- 1/4 teaspoon freshly ground black pepper

Step-by-Step Preparation Instructions:

1. In a large bowl, combine the drained and rinsed chickpeas, halved cherry tomatoes, diced cucumber, sliced red onion, crumbled feta cheese, and chopped fresh parsley.

2. In a small bowl, whisk together the lemon juice, olive oil, salt, and black pepper until well combined.

3. Drizzle the dressing over the chickpea

mixture and gently toss to coat all the ingredients evenly.

4. Adjust seasoning with additional salt and pepper if desired.

5. For an added flavor boost, you can incorporate a teaspoon of dried oregano or a minced garlic clove to the dressing.

6. Let the salad marinate for at least 30 minutes before serving to allow the flavors to meld together.

7. Serve chilled or at room temperature, garnished with extra parsley if desired.

Nutritional Information (per serving):

- Calories: 250
- Total Fat: 12g
- Saturated Fat: 3g
- Cholesterol: 10mg
- Sodium: 350mg
- Total Carbohydrates: 27g
- Dietary Fiber: 7g
- Protein: 9g

Dietary Recommendation

This Mediterranean Chickpea Salad is an excellent choice for those following a plant-based or vegetarian diet. It's rich in fiber, protein, and healthy fats from the chickpeas, olive oil, and feta cheese. The vibrant array of fresh vegetables and herbs provides a wealth of vitamins, minerals, and antioxidants.

For individuals with Myasthenia Gravis, this recipe can be a nourishing and gentle option. The chickpeas offer a good source of lean protein, while the vegetables and herbs contribute essential nutrients. The feta cheese provides a calcium boost, which can be beneficial for muscle function.

Grilled Chicken and Vegetable Wraps

Ingredients:

- 4 boneless, skinless chicken breasts
- 2 tablespoons olive oil
- 1 teaspoon dried oregano
- 1 teaspoon dried basil
- 1 teaspoon garlic powder
- Salt and black pepper, to taste
- 4 cups mixed greens (such as baby spinach, arugula, and romaine lettuce)
- 2 bell peppers (one red and one yellow), sliced
- 1 avocado, sliced
- 4 whole-wheat tortillas (8-inch)
- 1 cup tzatziki sauce (see recipe below)

For the Tzatziki Sauce:

- 1 cup plain Greek yogurt
- 1 cucumber, grated and drained
- 2 cloves garlic, minced
- 2 tablespoons lemon juice
- 2 tablespoons chopped fresh dill
- Salt and black pepper, to taste

Step-by-Step Preparation Instructions:

1. **Prepare the Chicken:** Preheat an outdoor grill or indoor grill pan to medium-high heat. Brush the chicken breasts with olive oil and season with oregano, basil, garlic powder, salt, and black pepper. Grill the chicken for about 6-8 minutes per side, or until cooked through and juices run clear. Let the grilled chicken rest for 5 minutes, then slice or chop into bite-sized pieces.

2. **Make the Tzatziki Sauce:** In a small bowl, combine the Greek yogurt, grated cucumber, minced garlic, lemon juice, and chopped dill. Season with salt and black pepper to taste. Mix well and refrigerate until ready to use.

3. **Assemble the Wraps:** Warm the whole-wheat tortillas according to package instructions or wrap them in a damp paper towel and microwave for 20-30 seconds. Place a handful of mixed greens on each tortilla, followed by slices of bell peppers, avocado, and the grilled chicken pieces. Drizzle a generous amount of

tzatziki sauce over the filling.

4. **Wrap and Serve:** Fold the bottom of the tortilla over the filling, then fold in the sides and roll it up tightly into a wrap. Serve the wraps with any remaining tzatziki sauce on the side for dipping.

Nutritional Information (per serving):

- Calories: 410
- Total Fat: 18g
- Saturated Fat: 3g
- Cholesterol: 70mg
- Sodium: 480mg
- Total Carbohydrates: 35g
- Dietary Fiber: 7g
- Protein: 30g

Dietary Recommendation

These grilled chicken and vegetable wraps are a nutritious and well-balanced meal choice that aligns with the "Dietary Guidelines for Americans." They provide a good source of lean protein from the grilled chicken, as well as a variety of vegetables, including mixed greens, bell peppers, and avocado, which contribute essential vitamins, minerals, and dietary fiber.

The whole-wheat tortillas offer a healthier alternative to regular flour tortillas, providing additional fiber and nutrients. The tzatziki sauce, made with Greek yogurt, cucumber, and fresh herbs, adds a refreshing and flavorful touch while providing a boost of probiotics.

To accommodate individuals with swallowing difficulties associated with myasthenia gravis, it is recommended to moisten the wrap filling with the tzatziki sauce or other dressings to make it easier to swallow. Additionally, you can chop or mince the ingredients into smaller pieces to reduce the risk of choking or aspiration.

For those with fatigue concerns, consider preparing the wrap ingredients in advance and assembling the wraps closer to mealtime to conserve energy. Alternatively, you can enjoy the ingredients as a salad or bowl instead of a wrap.

Quinoa and Black Bean Burrito Bowls

Ingredients:

- 1 cup uncooked quinoa
- 2 cups cooked black beans (or 1 15-oz can, drained and rinsed)
- 1 large tomato, diced
- 1 ripe avocado, diced
- 2 cups shredded lettuce
- 1 cup salsa (your preferred variety)
- 1 tablespoon olive oil

- 1 teaspoon cumin powder
- 1 teaspoon chili powder
- 1 teaspoon garlic powder
- Salt and pepper to taste
- Lime wedges for serving (optional)

Step-by-Step Preparation Instructions:

1. Rinse the quinoa thoroughly under cold water using a fine mesh strainer. Transfer the quinoa to a saucepan and add 2 cups of water or vegetable broth. Bring the mixture to a boil, then reduce the heat to low, cover, and simmer for 15-20 minutes, or until the quinoa is fluffy and the liquid is absorbed.

2. While the quinoa is cooking, prepare the other ingredients. In a large bowl, combine the cooked black beans, diced tomato, diced avocado, and shredded lettuce.

3. In a small bowl, mix together the olive oil, cumin powder, chili powder, garlic powder, salt, and pepper. This seasoning blend will add a burst of flavour to the quinoa and bean mixture.

4. Once the quinoa is cooked, fluff it with a fork and transfer it to the large bowl with the black bean mixture. Drizzle the seasoning blend over the quinoa and beans, and gently toss to combine all the ingredients.

5. To serve, divide the quinoa and black bean mixture evenly into serving bowls. Top each bowl with a generous spoonful of salsa. If

desired, garnish with lime wedges for an extra zing of flavour.

Nutritional Information (per serving):

- Calories: 320
- Protein: 12g
- Carbohydrates: 48g
- Fiber: 12g
- Fat: 10g
- Saturated Fat: 1.5g
- Sodium: 280mg

Dietary Recommendation

This quinoa and black bean burrito bowl is an excellent choice for those following a plant-based diet or looking for a nutrient-dense meal. Quinoa is a complete protein source, providing all nine essential amino acids, while black beans are rich in fiber, iron, and antioxidants.

This dish is also suitable for individuals with Myasthenia Gravis, as it is low in saturated fat and cholesterol, and the quinoa and black beans provide a good source of potassium, which is essential for proper muscle function.

To enhance the flavor and add a touch of creaminess, you can consider topping the burrito bowls with a dollop of plain Greek yogurt or a drizzle of tahini sauce. Additionally, you can incorporate fresh herbs like cilantro or parsley for an extra burst of flavor and nutrition.

Remember to chew the quinoa and black bean mixture thoroughly to aid in digestion and avoid any potential swallowing difficulties associated with Myasthenia Gravis.

Roasted Vegetable and Hummus Sandwich

Ingredients:

- 8 slices of whole-grain bread
- 1 cup of hummus
- 2 bell peppers (any color), sliced
- 1 zucchini, sliced into rounds
- 2 cups of mixed greens (arugula, spinach, romaine lettuce)
- 2 tablespoons of olive oil
- 1 teaspoon of dried oregano
- Salt and black pepper, to taste

Step-by-Step Preparation Instructions:

1. Preheat your oven to 400°F (200°C).

2. On a large baking sheet, arrange the sliced bell peppers and zucchini in a single layer. Drizzle with olive oil, oregano, salt, and black pepper. Toss to coat evenly.

3. Roast the vegetables in the preheated oven for 20-25 minutes, or until they are tender and slightly charred around the edges. Remove

from the oven and let cool slightly.

4. Toast the whole-grain bread slices until lightly browned.

5. Spread a generous amount of hummus on four slices of the toasted bread.

6. Top the hummus with the roasted vegetables, distributing them evenly over the four slices.

7. Arrange the mixed greens on top of the roasted vegetables.

8. Cover each sandwich with the remaining four slices of toasted bread.

9. Slice the sandwiches diagonally and serve immediately.

Flavor Enhancer (Optional): For an added burst of flavor, you can drizzle the roasted vegetables with a tablespoon of balsamic vinegar or lemon juice before assembling the sandwiches.

Nutritional Information (per sandwich):

- Calories: 380
- Total Fat: 16g
- Saturated Fat: 2g
- Cholesterol: 0mg
- Sodium: 390mg
- Total Carbohydrates: 48g
- Dietary Fiber: 9g
- Protein: 12g

Dietary Recommendation

This roasted vegetable and hummus sandwich is an excellent choice for those following a plant-based or vegetarian diet. It's packed with wholesome ingredients, including whole grains, vegetables, and protein-rich hummus. The roasted vegetables provide a delightful texture and flavor, while the mixed greens add freshness and crunch. This sandwich is also a great option for those looking to incorporate more fiber and nutrients into their diet.

Baked Cod with Tomato and Olive Sauce

Ingredients:

- 4 cod fillets (approximately 6 ounces each)
- 1 (14.5 oz) can of diced tomatoes
- 1/2 cup of Kalamata olives, pitted and halved
- 4 cloves of garlic, minced
- 2 tablespoons of olive oil
- 1/4 cup of fresh basil leaves, chopped
- Salt and black pepper, to taste

Step-by-Step Preparation Instructions:

1. Preheat your oven to 400°F (200°C).

2. In a shallow baking dish, arrange the cod fillets in a single layer.

3. In a separate bowl, combine the diced

tomatoes, Kalamata olives, minced garlic, olive oil, and chopped basil. Season with salt and black pepper to taste.

4. Pour the tomato and olive mixture over the cod fillets, ensuring they are evenly coated.

5. Cover the baking dish with aluminum foil and bake for 20-25 minutes, or until the cod is opaque and flakes easily with a fork.

6. Remove the foil and continue baking for an additional 5 minutes to allow the sauce to slightly thicken.

7. Serve the baked cod fillets hot, with the tomato and olive sauce spooned over the top.

Flavor Enhancer (Optional): For an extra kick of flavor, you can add a pinch of red pepper flakes or a squeeze of fresh lemon juice to the tomato and olive sauce before baking.

Nutritional Information (per serving):

- Calories: 280
- Total Fat: 12g
- Saturated Fat: 2g
- Cholesterol: 60mg
- Sodium: 480mg
- Total Carbohydrates: 8g
- Dietary Fiber: 2g
- Protein: 34g

Dietary Recommendation

This baked cod with tomato and olive sauce is an

excellent choice for those looking for a lean protein source with a burst of Mediterranean flavors. Cod is a low-calorie, high-protein fish that is also rich in essential nutrients like vitamin B12, selenium, and potassium. The tomato and olive sauce adds a flavorful twist, while the garlic and basil provide an aromatic depth.

Spinach and Feta Frittata

Ingredients:

- 8 large eggs
- 1 cup fresh spinach, roughly chopped
- 1/2 cup crumbled feta cheese
- 1/2 cup diced onions
- 1/2 cup cherry tomatoes, halved
- 2 tablespoons olive oil
- Salt and freshly ground black pepper, to taste

Step-by-Step Preparation Instructions:

1. Preheat your oven to 375°F (190°C).

2. In a medium-sized bowl, whisk the eggs together with a fork or whisk until well combined and slightly frothy.

3. Heat the olive oil in a 9-inch oven-safe skillet or cast-iron pan over medium heat.

4. Add the diced onions to the pan and sauté for 2-3 minutes until they become translucent and fragrant.

5. Add the chopped spinach to the pan and sauté for another minute or two until the spinach begins to wilt.

6. Pour the whisked eggs into the pan and distribute the spinach and onions evenly throughout the mixture.

7. Sprinkle the crumbled feta cheese and halved cherry tomatoes over the top of the frittata.

8. Transfer the skillet to the preheated oven and bake for 12-15 minutes, or until the frittata is set and the top is lightly golden brown.

9. Remove the frittata from the oven and let it cool for a few minutes before slicing and serving.

Flavor Enhancer: For an extra burst of flavor, you can add a pinch of dried herbs like thyme, oregano, or basil to the egg mixture before pouring it into the pan.

Nutritional Information (per serving):

- Calories: 210
- Protein: 14g
- Total Fat: 15g
- Saturated Fat: 5g
- Cholesterol: 285mg
- Total Carbohydrates: 4g
- Dietary Fiber: 1g
- Sodium: 280mg

Dietary Recommendation

This spinach and feta frittata is a delightful and nutritious option for any meal of the day. It's packed with protein from the eggs and feta cheese, as well as a generous serving of spinach, which provides valuable vitamins and minerals. The cherry tomatoes add a burst of freshness and a touch of sweetness to the dish.

This frittata is a great choice for those following a low-carb or high-protein diet, as it's relatively low in carbohydrates and rich in protein. Additionally, it's a versatile dish that can be enjoyed hot or cold, making it an excellent option for meal prepping or on-the-go snacking.

Grilled Chicken and Pineapple Skewers

Ingredients:

- 1 lb boneless, skinless chicken breasts, cut into 1-inch cubes
- 1 fresh pineapple, peeled, cored, and cut into 1-inch chunks
- 1 red bell pepper, cut into 1-inch pieces
- 1 green bell pepper, cut into 1-inch pieces
- 1/2 cup teriyaki sauce
- 2 tablespoons olive oil
- Salt and freshly ground black pepper, to taste
- Wooden skewers, soaked in water for at least 30 minutes

Step-by-Step Preparation Instructions:

1. In a large bowl, combine the cubed chicken, pineapple chunks, red and green bell pepper pieces, teriyaki sauce, and olive oil. Toss

well to coat the ingredients evenly with the teriyaki sauce.

2. Season the mixture with salt and black pepper to taste.

3. Thread the chicken, pineapple, and bell pepper pieces onto the soaked wooden skewers, alternating the ingredients for a visually appealing presentation.

4. Preheat your grill or grill pan to medium-high heat.

5. Grill the skewers for 12-15 minutes, turning occasionally, until the chicken is cooked through and the pineapple and bell peppers are slightly charred and tender.

6. Baste the skewers with any remaining teriyaki sauce from the bowl during the grilling process to enhance the flavor and create a delicious glaze.

7. Remove the skewers from the grill and let them rest for a few minutes before serving.

Flavor Enhancer: For an extra kick of flavor, consider adding a teaspoon of grated fresh ginger or a minced garlic clove to the teriyaki sauce mixture before marinating the ingredients.

Nutritional Information (per serving):

- Calories: 320
- Protein: 28g
- Total Fat: 8g
- Saturated Fat: 1g

- Cholesterol: 70mg
- Total Carbohydrates: 34g
- Dietary Fiber: 2g
- Sodium: 600mg

Dietary Recommendation

These grilled chicken and pineapple skewers are a delightful and healthy option for those seeking a flavorful and satisfying meal. The combination of lean chicken, juicy pineapple, and crunchy bell peppers provides a delightful medley of textures and flavors.

The teriyaki sauce adds a sweet and savory glaze to the skewers, making them a crowd-pleasing dish for any occasion. These skewers are an excellent source of protein from the chicken, as well as essential vitamins and minerals from the pineapple and bell peppers.

Lentil and Sweet Potato Shepherd's Pie

Ingredients:

- 1 cup dry green lentils
- 4 cups vegetable broth
- 2 large sweet potatoes, peeled and cubed
- 2 carrots, peeled and diced
- 1 cup frozen peas
- 1 onion, diced
- 3 cloves garlic, minced

- 2 tablespoons olive oil
- 1 teaspoon dried thyme
- Salt and pepper, to taste

Step-by-Step Preparation Instructions:

1. Preheat your oven to 375°F (190°C).

2. Rinse the lentils and place them in a saucepan with the vegetable broth. Bring to a boil, then reduce heat to low, cover, and simmer for 20-25 minutes, or until lentils are tender.

3. While the lentils are cooking, steam or boil the cubed sweet potatoes until fork-tender, about 10-15 minutes. Mash them with a fork or potato masher, and set aside.

4. In a skillet, heat the olive oil over medium heat. Add the diced onion and sauté for 2-3 minutes until translucent. Then, add the minced garlic and diced carrots, and sauté for another 2-3 minutes.

5. Drain any excess liquid from the cooked lentils and add them to the skillet with the onion, garlic, and carrots. Stir in the frozen peas, dried thyme, salt, and pepper. Mix well and remove from heat.

6. In a baking dish, spread the lentil mixture evenly on the bottom. Top with the mashed sweet potatoes, spreading them out to cover the lentil mixture completely.

7. Bake in the preheated oven for 25-30 minutes, or until the top is lightly browned.

8. **Flavor Enhancer:** For an extra depth of

flavor, consider adding a tablespoon of Dijon mustard or a splash of Worcestershire sauce to the lentil mixture before baking.

Nutritional Information (per serving):

- Calories: 250
- Total Fat: 5g
- Saturated Fat: 1g
- Cholesterol: 0mg
- Sodium: 200mg
- Total Carbohydrates: 40g
- Dietary Fiber: 10g
- Protein: 10g

Dietary Recommendation

This hearty and flavorful Lentil and Sweet Potato Shepherd's Pie is an excellent choice for those following a plant-based or vegetarian diet. It's packed with nutrients, including fiber, protein, and various vitamins and minerals. The combination of lentils and sweet potatoes provides a satisfying and filling meal, making it a great option for lunch or dinner.

Baked Salmon with Mango Salsa

Ingredients:

- 4 salmon fillets (6-8 ounces each)
- 2 tablespoons olive oil
- Salt and pepper, to taste

For the Mango Salsa:

- 2 ripe mangoes, diced
- 1/2 red onion, finely diced
- 1/4 cup chopped fresh cilantro
- 1 jalapeño, seeds removed and finely diced
- Juice of 1 lime
- Salt and pepper, to taste

Step-by-Step Preparation Instructions:

1. Preheat your oven to 400°F (200°C).

2. Prepare the mango salsa by combining the diced mangoes, red onion, cilantro, jalapeño, lime juice, salt, and pepper in a bowl. Mix well and set aside.

3. Place the salmon fillets on a baking sheet lined with parchment paper or a silicone mat. Brush the fillets with olive oil and season with salt and pepper.

4. Bake the salmon for 12-15 minutes, or until it flakes easily with a fork and is cooked through.

5. Remove the salmon from the oven and let it rest for 5 minutes.

6. Serve the baked salmon fillets warm, topped with a generous portion of the refreshing mango salsa.

Nutritional Information (per serving):

- Calories: 350
- Total Fat: 18g

- Saturated Fat: 3g
- Cholesterol: 90mg
- Sodium: 120mg
- Total Carbohydrates: 15g
- Dietary Fiber: 2g
- Protein: 35g

Dietary Recommendation

This Baked Salmon with Mango Salsa is an excellent choice for those looking for a lean protein option with a burst of fresh flavors. Salmon is rich in heart-healthy omega-3 fatty acids, while the mango salsa provides a vibrant and refreshing contrast to the rich fish.

Greek Quinoa Salad

Ingredients:

- 1 cup quinoa, rinsed and cooked according to package instructions
- 1 cup cherry tomatoes, halved
- 1 English cucumber, diced
- 1/2 red onion, thinly sliced
- 1/2 cup crumbled feta cheese
- 1/2 cup Kalamata olives, pitted and halved
- 1/4 cup extra virgin olive oil
- 2 tablespoons red wine vinegar
- 1 tablespoon fresh lemon juice
- 1 teaspoon dried oregano

- 1/2 teaspoon salt
- 1/4 teaspoon black pepper

Step-by-Step Preparation Instructions:

1. Cook the quinoa according to package instructions. Once cooked, fluff with a fork and allow to cool slightly.

2. In a large bowl, combine the cooked and cooled quinoa, cherry tomatoes, cucumber, red onion, feta cheese, and Kalamata olives. Gently toss to mix.

3. In a small bowl, whisk together the olive oil, red wine vinegar, lemon juice, oregano, salt, and black pepper to make the dressing.

4. Pour the dressing over the quinoa salad and toss gently to coat all ingredients evenly.

5. Cover the salad and refrigerate for at least 30 minutes to allow the flavors to meld.

6. Before serving, give the salad a gentle toss and adjust seasoning if needed. Garnish with extra feta cheese and olives if desired.

Flavor Enhancer (Optional): For an added depth of flavor, you can incorporate fresh herbs like parsley, mint, or dill into the salad. Additionally, you could add a pinch of red pepper flakes for a hint of heat.

Nutritional Information (per serving):

- Calories: 280
- Total Fat: 18g
- Saturated Fat: 4g

- Cholesterol: 15mg
- Sodium: 450mg
- Total Carbohydrates: 24g
- Dietary Fiber: 4g
- Sugars: 3g
- Protein: 8g

Dietary Recommendation

This Greek Quinoa Salad is a delightful and nutritious option for those following a Myasthenia Gravis diet. Quinoa is a gluten-free whole grain packed with protein, fiber, and essential nutrients, making it an excellent choice for promoting muscle strength and overall well-being.

The vibrant combination of fresh vegetables, including tomatoes, cucumber, and red onion, provides a rich array of vitamins, minerals, and antioxidants to support a healthy immune system. The addition of feta cheese contributes calcium and protein, while the Kalamata olives offer a burst of flavor and beneficial monounsaturated fats.

This salad can be enjoyed as a light main course or a nutritious side dish. Its versatility allows you to adjust the portions to suit your personal dietary needs and preferences.

Grilled Chicken and Vegetable Kebabs with Tzatziki Sauce

Ingredients:

For the Kebabs:

- 1 1/2 pounds boneless, skinless chicken breasts, cut into 1-inch cubes
- 2 bell peppers (red and yellow), cut into 1-inch pieces
- 2 zucchini, sliced into 1/2-inch rounds
- 1 red onion, cut into 1-inch pieces
- 1/4 cup olive oil
- 2 tablespoons lemon juice
- 2 cloves garlic, minced
- 1 teaspoon dried oregano
- 1/2 teaspoon salt
- 1/4 teaspoon black pepper

For the Tzatziki Sauce:

- 1 cup plain Greek yogurt
- 1/2 cucumber, grated and drained
- 2 cloves garlic, minced
- 2 tablespoons fresh dill, chopped
- 1 tablespoon lemon juice
- 1/2 teaspoon salt
- 1/4 teaspoon black pepper

Step-by-Step Preparation Instructions:

1. Prepare the Kebabs: a. In a large bowl, combine the cubed chicken, bell peppers, zucchini, and red onion. b. In a small bowl, whisk together the olive oil, lemon juice,

minced garlic, oregano, salt, and black pepper. c. Pour the marinade over the chicken and vegetable mixture, and toss to coat evenly. d. Cover and refrigerate for at least 30 minutes, or up to 2 hours, to allow the flavors to meld.

2. Prepare the Tzatziki Sauce: a. In a medium bowl, combine the Greek yogurt, grated cucumber, minced garlic, fresh dill, lemon juice, salt, and black pepper. b. Mix well and refrigerate until ready to serve.

3. Preheat an outdoor grill or indoor grill pan to medium-high heat.

4. Thread the marinated chicken, bell peppers, zucchini, and red onion onto metal or wooden skewers, alternating the ingredients.

5. Grill the kebabs for 12-15 minutes, rotating occasionally, until the chicken is cooked through and the vegetables are tender and charred in spots.

6. Transfer the grilled kebabs to a serving platter and serve with the chilled Tzatziki Sauce on the side for dipping or drizzling.

Nutritional Information (per serving):

- Calories: 310
- Total Fat: 14g
- Saturated Fat: 3g
- Cholesterol: 75mg
- Sodium: 590mg
- Total Carbohydrates: 16g
- Dietary Fiber: 3g

- Sugars: 7g
- Protein: 32g

Dietary Recommendation

These Grilled Chicken and Vegetable Kebabs with Tzatziki Sauce are an excellent choice for those following a Myasthenia Gravis diet. The lean protein from the chicken and the array of colorful vegetables provide a well-balanced meal rich in essential nutrients.

The marinade infuses the chicken and vegetables with a delightful blend of flavors, while the Tzatziki Sauce, made with Greek yogurt, cucumber, and fresh herbs, offers a refreshing and cooling accompaniment. This dish can be enjoyed as a main course or paired with a side of whole grains or a fresh salad for a complete and satisfying meal.

Baked Sweet Potato Fries with Garlic Aioli

Ingredients:

For the Sweet Potato Fries:

- 3 large sweet potatoes, peeled and cut into 1/2-inch thick fries
- 2 tablespoons olive oil
- 1 teaspoon smoked paprika
- 1/2 teaspoon garlic powder
- 1/2 teaspoon salt
- 1/4 teaspoon black pepper

For the Garlic Aioli:

- 1/2 cup mayonnaise
- 2 cloves garlic, minced
- 1 tablespoon lemon juice
- 1/4 teaspoon salt
- 1/8 teaspoon black pepper

Step-by-Step Preparation Instructions:

1. Preheat your oven to 425°F (220°C). Line a large baking sheet with parchment paper.

2. In a large bowl, toss the cut sweet potato fries with olive oil, smoked paprika, garlic powder, salt, and black pepper until evenly coated.

3. Spread the seasoned fries in a single layer on the prepared baking sheet, ensuring they are not overcrowded.

4. Bake for 20 minutes, then flip the fries with a spatula and bake for an additional 10-15 minutes, or until the fries are golden brown and crispy.

5. While the fries are baking, prepare the garlic aioli by mixing together the mayonnaise, minced garlic, lemon juice, salt, and black pepper in a small bowl.

6. Once the fries are done, transfer them to a serving platter and serve hot with the garlic aioli on the side for dipping.

Flavor Enhancer (Optional): For an extra burst of flavor, consider sprinkling the baked fries with fresh herbs like chopped parsley or cilantro before serving.

Nutritional Information (per serving):

- Calories: 280
- Total Fat: 18g
- Saturated Fat: 2.5g
- Cholesterol: 10mg
- Sodium: 540mg
- Total Carbohydrates: 27g
- Dietary Fiber: 4g
- Sugars: 6g
- Protein: 3g

Dietary Recommendation

These baked sweet potato fries are a healthier alternative to traditional fried french fries, as they are baked instead of fried, reducing the overall fat content. Sweet potatoes are an excellent source of vitamins A and C, as well as dietary fiber, making this dish a nutrient-dense choice.

The garlic aioli adds a creamy and flavorful dipping sauce, but be mindful of portion control as it contains mayonnaise, which can contribute to higher saturated fat and calorie intake. To incorporate more lean protein, consider pairing these fries with grilled chicken or fish. For a vegetarian option, you can serve them alongside a lentil or bean-based dish.

Vegetable and Tofu Stir-Fry with Brown Rice Noodles

Ingredients:

- 1 package (14 oz) extra-firm tofu, drained and cut into 1-inch cubes
- 2 tablespoons olive oil, divided
- 1 cup broccoli florets
- 1 cup sliced carrots
- 1 red bell pepper, sliced
- 2 cloves garlic, minced
- 1 tablespoon grated fresh ginger
- 1/4 cup low-sodium soy sauce
- 1 tablespoon rice vinegar
- 1 teaspoon sesame oil
- 8 oz brown rice noodles, cooked according to package instructions
- 2 green onions, sliced (for garnish)

Step-by-Step Preparation Instructions:

1. In a large skillet or wok, heat 1 tablespoon of olive oil over medium-high heat. Add the tofu cubes and cook for 5-7 minutes, stirring occasionally, until lightly browned on all sides. Transfer the cooked tofu to a plate and set aside.

2. In the same skillet or wok, heat the remaining 1 tablespoon of olive oil. Add the broccoli, carrots, and bell pepper. Stir-fry for 3-4 minutes until the vegetables are slightly tender but still crisp.

3. Add the minced garlic and grated ginger to the skillet or wok, and stir-fry for another minute until fragrant.

4. Pour in the low-sodium soy sauce, rice vinegar, and sesame oil. Stir to combine and allow the sauce to simmer for 1-2 minutes.

5. Return the cooked tofu to the skillet or wok, along with the cooked brown rice noodles. Gently toss everything together until the noodles and tofu are well coated with the sauce.

6. Remove from heat and garnish with sliced green onions.

7. Serve hot and enjoy!

Nutritional Information (per serving):

- Calories: 350
- Total Fat: 12g
- Saturated Fat: 1.5g
- Cholesterol: 0mg
- Sodium: 600mg
- Total Carbohydrates: 50g
- Dietary Fiber: 6g
- Sugars: 5g
- Protein: 15g

Dietary Recommendation

This vegetable and tofu stir-fry is a well-balanced and nutritious meal that incorporates lean protein from tofu, fiber-rich vegetables, and whole-grain brown rice noodles. It is low in saturated fat and cholesterol, making it a heart-healthy option.

To further enhance the nutritional value, consider

adding more vegetables like mushrooms, snow peas, or bean sprouts. You can also adjust the amount of soy sauce to reduce sodium intake if desired. For those following a gluten-free diet, ensure that the soy sauce and brown rice noodles used are gluten-free varieties.

Grilled Salmon and Asparagus Salad with Lemon Vinaigrette

Ingredients:

For the Salad:

- 4 (6-ounce) salmon fillets
- 1 bunch asparagus, trimmed
- 8 cups mixed greens (such as arugula, spinach, and romaine)
- 1 cup cherry tomatoes, halved

For the Lemon Vinaigrette:

- 1/4 cup freshly squeezed lemon juice
- 2 tablespoons white wine vinegar
- 1 tablespoon Dijon mustard
- 1 garlic clove, minced
- 1/2 cup extra-virgin olive oil
- Salt and freshly ground black pepper, to taste

Step-by-Step Preparation Instructions:

1. Preheat an outdoor grill or grill pan to medium-high heat.

2. Brush the salmon fillets and asparagus with a light coating of olive oil and season with salt and pepper.

3. Grill the salmon until cooked through, about 4-6 minutes per side, depending on thickness. Transfer to a plate and let cool slightly.

4. Grill the asparagus until tender-crisp, about 3-4 minutes, turning occasionally. Remove from the grill and let cool slightly.

5. In a small bowl, whisk together the lemon juice, vinegar, mustard, and garlic. Slowly drizzle in the olive oil while whisking continuously until the vinaigrette is emulsified. Season with salt and pepper to taste.

6. In a large salad bowl, combine the mixed greens, cherry tomatoes, grilled salmon (flaked into large chunks), and grilled asparagus.

7. Drizzle the lemon vinaigrette over the salad and toss gently to coat.

8. Serve the salad immediately, garnished with additional lemon wedges, if desired.

Nutritional Information (per serving):

- Calories: 420
- Total Fat: 28g
- Saturated Fat: 4g
- Cholesterol: 65mg
- Sodium: 220mg
- Total Carbohydrates: 12g

- Dietary Fiber: 4g
- Protein: 32g

Dietary Recommendation

This salad is an excellent choice for those following a balanced, nutrient-dense diet. It offers a harmonious blend of lean protein from the grilled salmon, fiber-rich vegetables, and a tangy, flavorful dressing made with heart-healthy olive oil. The asparagus and mixed greens provide valuable vitamins, minerals, and antioxidants, while the lemon vinaigrette adds a refreshing zing to the dish.

Quinoa and Black Bean Stuffed Bell Peppers

Ingredients:

- 4 large bell peppers (any color), halved lengthwise and seeded
- 1 cup uncooked quinoa, rinsed
- 1 (15-ounce) can black beans, drained and rinsed
- 1 (14.5-ounce) can diced tomatoes
- 1 small onion, diced
- 3 garlic cloves, minced
- 1 teaspoon ground cumin
- 1/2 teaspoon chili powder (optional)
- 1/4 cup fresh cilantro, chopped
- Salt and freshly ground black pepper, to taste

- 1/2 cup shredded cheese (such as cheddar or Mexican blend), for topping (optional)

Step-by-Step Preparation Instructions:

1. Preheat your oven to 375°F (190°C).

2. Cook the quinoa according to package instructions. Fluff with a fork and set aside to cool slightly.

3. In a large skillet, sauté the onion and garlic in a tablespoon of olive oil over medium heat until translucent, about 3-4 minutes.

4. Add the diced tomatoes (with their juices), black beans, cumin, chili powder (if using), and salt and pepper to taste. Stir to combine and cook for 2-3 minutes.

5. Remove the skillet from heat and stir in the cooked quinoa and chopped cilantro.

6. Place the bell pepper halves in a baking dish or on a rimmed baking sheet.

7. Spoon the quinoa and black bean mixture into the bell pepper halves, filling them generously.

8. If desired, top the stuffed peppers with shredded cheese.

9. Cover the baking dish or baking sheet with aluminum foil and bake for 30 minutes.

10. Remove the foil and bake for an additional 10-15 minutes, or until the peppers are tender and the cheese (if using) is melted and bubbly.

11. Serve the stuffed bell peppers warm, garnished with additional chopped cilantro, if desired.

Nutritional Information (per serving, without cheese):

- Calories: 290
- Total Fat: 4g
- Saturated Fat: 0.5g
- Cholesterol: 0mg
- Sodium: 280mg
- Total Carbohydrates: 52g
- Dietary Fiber: 13g
- Protein: 13g

Dietary Recommendation

These quinoa and black bean stuffed bell peppers are a nutritious and satisfying vegetarian meal option. Quinoa provides a complete protein source, while black beans contribute additional protein and fiber. The bell peppers are an excellent source of vitamins A and C, as well as antioxidants. This dish is suitable for those following a plant-based or gluten-free diet.

Baked Chicken with Roasted Brussels Sprouts and Sweet Potatoes

Ingredients:

- 4 boneless, skinless chicken breasts
- 1 pound Brussels sprouts, trimmed and halved
- 2 medium sweet potatoes, peeled and cut into 1-inch cubes
- 4 tablespoons olive oil, divided
- 3 garlic cloves, minced
- 1 tablespoon fresh rosemary, chopped
- 1 teaspoon fresh thyme leaves
- Salt and freshly ground black pepper, to taste

Step-by-Step Preparation Instructions:

1. Preheat your oven to 400°F (200°C).

2. In a large bowl, toss the Brussels sprouts and sweet potato cubes with 2 tablespoons of olive oil, garlic, rosemary, thyme, salt, and pepper. Spread the vegetable mixture evenly on a large rimmed baking sheet.

3. Place the chicken breasts on the same baking sheet, spaced apart from the vegetables. Brush or drizzle the remaining 2 tablespoons of olive oil over the chicken breasts, and season with salt and pepper.

4. Roast in the preheated oven for 25-30 minutes, or until the chicken is cooked through (internal temperature reaches 165°F/74°C) and the vegetables are tender and caramelized.

5. Remove the baking sheet from the oven and let the chicken and vegetables rest for 5 minutes before serving.

Nutritional Information (per serving):

- Calories: 450
- Total Fat: 16g
- Saturated Fat: 2.5g
- Cholesterol: 105mg
- Sodium: 280mg
- Total Carbohydrates: 35g
- Dietary Fiber: 6g
- Protein: 42g

Vegetable and Lentil Soup with Pesto

Ingredients:

- 1 cup dried lentils (green or brown)
- 1 (14.5 oz) can diced tomatoes
- 3 carrots, peeled and diced
- 3 celery stalks, diced
- 1 onion, diced
- 4 cloves garlic, minced
- 6 cups vegetable or chicken broth
- 1 bay leaf
- 1 tsp dried thyme
- Salt and freshly ground black pepper, to taste
- 2 cups baby spinach or kale, chopped
- 1/4 cup fresh basil pesto (homemade or store-bought)

For the Basil Pesto:

- 2 cups fresh basil leaves
- 1/4 cup pine nuts or walnuts
- 2 garlic cloves
- 1/2 cup grated Parmesan cheese
- 1/2 cup extra-virgin olive oil
- Salt and pepper, to taste

Step-by-Step Preparation Instructions:

1. Rinse the lentils under cold water and pick out any debris or stones. Set aside.

2. In a large pot or Dutch oven, sauté the diced onion and garlic in a tablespoon of olive oil over medium heat until fragrant, about 2 minutes.

3. Add the diced carrots, celery, diced tomatoes with their juices, lentils, broth, bay leaf, thyme, salt, and pepper. Stir to combine.

4. Bring the mixture to a boil, then reduce heat to low, cover, and simmer for 20-25 minutes, or until the lentils and vegetables are tender.

5. While the soup is simmering, prepare the basil pesto. In a food processor, combine the basil leaves, pine nuts (or walnuts), garlic cloves, Parmesan cheese, olive oil, salt, and pepper. Pulse until the mixture forms a coarse paste. Adjust seasoning to taste.

6. Once the soup is ready, remove the bay leaf. Stir in the chopped spinach or kale and let it wilt for a minute or two.

7. Ladle the soup into bowls and swirl a dollop of fresh basil pesto into each serving.

Nutritional Information (per serving):

- Calories: 320
- Total Fat: 15g
- Saturated Fat: 2g
- Cholesterol: 5mg
- Sodium: 650mg
- Total Carbohydrates: 35g
- Dietary Fiber: 13g
- Protein: 15g

Dietary Recommendation

This hearty and flavorful vegetable and lentil soup is an excellent source of plant-based protein, fiber, and various essential vitamins and minerals. The addition of basil pesto adds a burst of fresh, herbaceous flavor and a touch of healthy fats.

This soup is suitable for vegetarians and can be made vegan by omitting the Parmesan cheese in the pesto or using a vegan alternative. It's also low in saturated fat and cholesterol, making it a heart-healthy option. Lentils are an excellent choice for those with myasthenia gravis, as they are easy to chew and swallow, and provide a good source of energy and nutrients without being overly taxing on the digestive system.

Mediterranean Chickpea Salad with Grilled Shrimp

Ingredients:

- 1 can (15 oz) chickpeas, drained and rinsed
- 1 pint cherry tomatoes, halved
- 1 cucumber, diced
- 1/2 red onion, finely chopped
- 1/2 cup crumbled feta cheese
- 1/4 cup chopped fresh parsley
- 2 tbsp freshly squeezed lemon juice
- 2 tbsp extra virgin olive oil
- Salt and freshly ground black pepper, to taste
- 1 lb large shrimp, peeled and deveined
- 1 tsp dried oregano
- 1 garlic clove, minced

Preparation:

1. In a large bowl, combine the chickpeas, cherry tomatoes, cucumber, red onion, feta cheese, and parsley. Gently toss to combine.

2. In a small bowl, whisk together the lemon juice, 1 tablespoon of the olive oil, salt, and pepper. Drizzle the dressing over the salad and toss to coat evenly. Set aside.

3. In a separate bowl, combine the shrimp, remaining 1 tablespoon of olive oil, oregano, garlic, salt, and pepper. Toss to coat the

shrimp thoroughly.

4. Heat a grill pan or outdoor grill over medium-high heat. Once hot, add the marinated shrimp and cook for 2-3 minutes per side, until they turn pink and are cooked through.

5. Arrange the grilled shrimp on top of the chickpea salad. For added flavor, squeeze a bit of lemon juice over the shrimp before serving.

6. Serve the Mediterranean Chickpea Salad with Grilled Shrimp immediately, either on individual plates or in a large serving bowl for family-style dining. Enjoy this refreshing and nourishing meal!

Nutritional Information (per serving, based on 4 servings):

- Calories: 365
- Total Fat: 16g
- Saturated Fat: 5g
- Cholesterol: 179mg
- Sodium: 648mg
- Total Carbohydrates: 27g
- Dietary Fiber: 8g
- Sugars: 6g
- Protein: 31g

Dietary Recommendations

This Mediterranean Chickpea Salad with Grilled Shrimp is an ideal dish for those following the dietary guidelines recommended for individuals with Myasthenia Gravis.

The salad is packed with nutrient-rich ingredients like chickpeas, vegetables, and lean protein from the shrimp. The dressing is made with heart-healthy olive oil and freshly squeezed lemon juice, providing a flavorful and refreshing taste without the need for excessive salt or sugar.

To make this dish even more MG-friendly, consider chopping the vegetables into smaller pieces for easier chewing and swallowing. The softness of the chickpeas and the tenderness of the grilled shrimp also make this salad a great option for those experiencing difficulty with solid foods.

Quinoa and Roasted Vegetable Grain Bowls

Ingredients:

- 1 cup uncooked quinoa, rinsed
- 2 cups water or low-sodium vegetable broth
- 2 cups broccoli florets
- 2 cups cauliflower florets
- 1 red bell pepper, sliced
- 1 yellow bell pepper, sliced
- 2 tbsp extra virgin olive oil
- 3 garlic cloves, minced
- 1/2 tsp salt
- 1/4 tsp freshly ground black pepper
- 2 tbsp freshly squeezed lemon juice

- 1/4 cup crumbled feta cheese (optional)
- Fresh parsley, chopped (for garnish)

Preparation:

1. Preheat the oven to 425°F (220°C). Line a large baking sheet with parchment paper.

2. In a medium saucepan, combine the rinsed quinoa and water (or vegetable broth). Bring the mixture to a boil, then reduce the heat to low, cover, and simmer for 15-20 minutes, or until the quinoa is tender and the liquid is absorbed. Remove from heat, fluff with a fork, and set aside.

3. In a large bowl, toss the broccoli, cauliflower, and sliced bell peppers with 1 tablespoon of olive oil, minced garlic, salt, and pepper until evenly coated.

4. Spread the seasoned vegetables in a single layer on the prepared baking sheet. Roast in the preheated oven for 20-25 minutes, or until the vegetables are tender and lightly caramelized, stirring halfway through.

5. In a small bowl, whisk together the remaining 1 tablespoon of olive oil and lemon juice to create a simple dressing.

6. Divide the cooked quinoa evenly among 4 serving bowls. Top each bowl with the roasted vegetables, then drizzle the lemon dressing over the top.

7. If desired, sprinkle crumbled feta cheese over each bowl for added creaminess and flavor.

8. Garnish with chopped fresh parsley and serve the Quinoa and Roasted Vegetable Grain Bowls warm.

Nutritional Information (per serving, based on 4 servings):

- Calories: 295
- Total Fat: 11g
- Saturated Fat: 2g
- Cholesterol: 0mg (without feta) or 8mg (with feta)
- Sodium: 375mg
- Total Carbohydrates: 42g
- Dietary Fiber: 7g
- Sugars: 4g
- Protein: 10g

Dietary Recommendations

These Quinoa and Roasted Vegetable Grain Bowls are a nutritious and delicious option for those following a diet tailored to manage Myasthenia Gravis symptoms. Quinoa is a nutrient-dense, gluten-free grain that provides essential amino acids, fiber, and minerals. The roasted vegetables offer a variety of vitamins, antioxidants, and fiber, which are important for overall health and well-being. The vegetables in this recipe are cooked until tender, making them easier to chew and swallow for individuals experiencing MG-related difficulties. The lemon dressing adds a bright, fresh flavor without relying on excessive salt or sugar.

Baked Cod with Tomato and Olive Tapenade

Ingredients:

- 4 (6-oz) cod fillets
- 1 (14.5-oz) can diced tomatoes, drained
- 1/2 cup pitted Kalamata olives, chopped
- 2 cloves garlic, minced
- 2 tablespoons olive oil
- 1/4 cup fresh basil leaves, chopped
- 2 tablespoons capers, drained

Preparation Instructions:

1. Preheat the oven to 400°F (200°C).

2. In a bowl, mix together the drained tomatoes, chopped olives, minced garlic, olive oil, chopped basil, and capers. Season with salt and pepper to taste.

3. Place the cod fillets in a baking dish. Spoon the tomato and olive mixture evenly over the top of each fillet.

4. Bake for 15-20 minutes, or until the fish is cooked through and easily flakes with a fork.

5. Serve the baked cod hot, garnished with additional fresh basil if desired.

Nutritional Information (per serving):

- Calories: 220
- Fat: 10g

- Saturated Fat: 1.5g
- Cholesterol: 60mg
- Sodium: 520mg
- Carbohydrates: 5g
- Fiber: 1g
- Sugar: 2g
- Protein: 28g

Dietary Recommendation:

This baked cod recipe is an excellent choice for those following a myasthenia gravis diet. Cod is a lean protein that is easy to chew and swallow, making it suitable for individuals who experience difficulty with these functions. The tomato and olive tapenade adds flavor and moisture to the dish, further aiding in ease of consumption.

Spinach and Feta Stuffed Chicken Breasts

Ingredients:

- 4 boneless, skinless chicken breasts
- 4 cups fresh spinach, chopped
- 1/2 cup crumbled feta cheese
- 1/4 cup onions, finely chopped
- 2 cloves garlic, minced
- 2 tablespoons olive oil
- Salt and pepper to taste

Preparation Instructions:

1. Preheat the oven to 375°F (190°C).

2. In a large skillet, heat the olive oil over medium heat. Add the chopped onions and minced garlic, and sauté until softened and fragrant, about 3-4 minutes.

3. Add the chopped spinach to the skillet and cook until wilted, about 2-3 minutes. Remove from heat and let cool slightly.

4. In a bowl, mix together the cooked spinach mixture and crumbled feta cheese. Season with salt and pepper to taste.

5. Cut a horizontal slit in each chicken breast to create a pocket. Stuff each pocket with the spinach and feta mixture, dividing it evenly among the breasts.

6. Place the stuffed chicken breasts in a baking dish. Brush with additional olive oil and season with salt and pepper.

7. Bake for 25-30 minutes, or until the chicken is cooked through and no longer pink in the center.

8. Serve the stuffed chicken breasts hot, garnished with additional feta cheese if desired.

Nutritional Information (per serving):

- Calories: 320
- Fat: 16g
- Saturated Fat: 5g

- Cholesterol: 110mg
- Sodium: 480mg
- Carbohydrates: 4g
- Fiber: 1g
- Sugar: 1g
- Protein: 38g

Dietary Recommendation:

These spinach and feta stuffed chicken breasts are a nutritious and flavorful option for those following a myasthenia gravis diet. The combination of lean protein from the chicken and nutrient-rich spinach helps to support overall health and well-being. The feta cheese adds moisture and flavor to the dish, making it easier to chew and swallow for those with muscle weakness.

Grilled Veggie and Hummus Wraps

Ingredients:

- 4 whole-wheat tortillas
- 1 cup hummus
- 1 zucchini, sliced lengthwise
- 1 red bell pepper, sliced
- 1 yellow bell pepper, sliced
- 1 onion, sliced into rings

- 2 cups mixed greens
- Salt and pepper to taste
- Olive oil for grilling

Instructions:

1. Preheat your grill or grill pan to medium-high heat. Brush the sliced zucchini, bell peppers, and onion with olive oil and season with salt and pepper.

2. Grill the vegetables for 3-4 minutes per side until they are tender and have nice grill marks. Remove from the grill and set aside.

3. Warm the whole-wheat tortillas on the grill for about 30 seconds per side, until they are pliable.

4. To assemble the wraps, spread 1/4 cup of hummus down the center of each tortilla. Top with the grilled vegetables and a handful of mixed greens.

5. Fold the sides of the tortilla over the filling, then roll tightly to form a wrap. Slice in half diagonally and serve immediately.

Nutritional Information (per serving):

- Calories: 290
- Fat: 11g
- Saturated Fat: 1.5g
- Carbohydrates: 38g
- Fiber: 8g
- Protein: 10g

Dietary Recommendations

These Grilled Veggie and Hummus Wraps are a nutritious and satisfying choice for those following a plant-based or vegetarian diet. The whole-wheat tortillas provide a good source of fiber, while the hummus offers protein and healthy fats. The grilled vegetables add a variety of vitamins, minerals, and antioxidants.

For an extra flavor boost, try brushing the vegetables with a mix of olive oil, lemon juice, minced garlic, and dried herbs like oregano or thyme before grilling. You can also experiment with different flavors of hummus, such as roasted red pepper or garlic, for added depth and interest. This recipe is easily adaptable to your preferences and can be made with any combination of your favorite grilled vegetables. It's perfect for a light lunch or dinner and can be prepared in advance for a quick and healthy meal on the go.

Sweet Potato and Black Bean Burrito Bowls

Ingredients:

- 2 large sweet potatoes, diced
- 1 tablespoon olive oil

- Salt and pepper to taste
- 1 can (15 oz) black beans, drained and rinsed
- 2 cups cooked brown rice
- 1 avocado, sliced
- 1/2 cup salsa
- Juice of 1 lime
- Optional toppings: cilantro, jalapeños, shredded cheese

Instructions:

1. Preheat your oven to 425°F (220°C). On a baking sheet, toss the diced sweet potatoes with olive oil, salt, and pepper. Roast for 25-30 minutes, stirring halfway through, until the sweet potatoes are tender and lightly caramelized.

2. In a small saucepan, heat the black beans over medium heat until warmed through. Season with salt and pepper to taste.

3. To assemble the burrito bowls, divide the cooked brown rice between four bowls. Top each bowl with equal amounts of the roasted sweet potatoes, black beans, sliced avocado, and salsa.

4. Squeeze fresh lime juice over each bowl and add any optional toppings as desired.

5. Serve the burrito bowls immediately while the ingredients are still warm.

Nutritional Information (per serving):

- Calories: 400

- Fat: 14g
- Saturated Fat: 2g
- Carbohydrates: 61g
- Fiber: 13g
- Protein: 12g

Dietary Recommendations

These Sweet Potato and Black Bean Burrito Bowls are a hearty and nutritious meal that is suitable for a variety of dietary needs. The combination of whole grains, legumes, and vegetables provides a balance of complex carbohydrates, plant-based protein, and healthy fats. Sweet potatoes are an excellent source of vitamin A, which supports eye health and immune function. Black beans are rich in fiber, protein, and various minerals like iron and magnesium. The addition of avocado provides heart-healthy monounsaturated fats and helps to keep you feeling full and satisfied.

Feel free to customize this recipe with your favorite burrito bowl toppings, such as grilled corn, diced tomatoes, or a dollop of plain Greek yogurt for added protein. You can also adjust the spice level by choosing a milder or hotter salsa based on your preferences. This dish is perfect for meal prepping and can be easily packed for a nutritious lunch at work or school. The leftovers can be stored in the refrigerator for up to 3-4 days, making it a convenient option for busy weeknights.

Lentil and Vegetable Curry with Coconut Milk

Ingredients:

- 1 cup red lentils, rinsed
- 1 can (400ml) coconut milk
- 1 can (400g) diced tomatoes
- 1 onion, diced
- 3 cloves garlic, minced
- 1 tbsp grated fresh ginger
- 2 tsp curry powder
- 2 cups mixed vegetables (such as carrots, peas, and spinach)
- Salt and pepper to taste
- Fresh cilantro for garnish

Preparation:

1. In a large pot, sauté the onion in a little oil over medium heat until translucent, about 5 minutes. Add the garlic and ginger and cook for another minute until fragrant.

2. Stir in the curry powder and cook for 30 seconds to release the spices' aroma. Pour in the diced tomatoes with their juices and the coconut milk. Bring the mixture to a simmer.

3. Add the rinsed red lentils to the pot. Cover and let simmer for 15 minutes, stirring occasionally.

4. Mix in the vegetables and continue simmering uncovered for another 10

minutes, or until the lentils and vegetables are tender. Season with salt and pepper to taste.

5. Serve the curry hot over rice or with naan bread if desired. Garnish with fresh cilantro for added flavor and visual appeal.

Nutritional Information (per serving):

- Calories: 320
- Fat: 14g
- Saturated Fat: 11g
- Carbohydrates: 38g
- Fiber: 18g
- Protein: 15g

Dietary Recommendations

This hearty lentil and vegetable curry is an excellent option for those with myasthenia gravis. Lentils provide a good source of plant-based protein that is easier to chew and swallow compared to tougher meats. The vegetables offer essential nutrients and the coconut milk adds healthy fats.

The soft texture of this curry makes it easier to eat for those experiencing chewing and swallowing difficulties. You can adjust the consistency by adding more liquid if needed. The warm spices like ginger and curry powder not only enhance the flavor but may also have anti-inflammatory properties. Feel free to modify the vegetables based on your preferences and what you have on hand. Serve with soft, well-cooked rice for a complete meal that is both delicious and myasthenia gravis-friendly.

Baked Salmon with Mango Salsa and Quinoa

Ingredients:

- 4 salmon fillets (4-6 oz each)
- 1 mango, diced
- 1/2 red onion, finely diced
- 1/4 cup chopped fresh cilantro
- Juice of 1 lime
- 1 jalapeño, seeded and minced (optional)
- 1 cup cooked quinoa
- Salt and pepper
- Olive oil

Preparation:

1. Preheat the oven to 400°F (200°C). Line a baking sheet with parchment paper.

2. Season the salmon fillets with salt and pepper and place them on the prepared baking sheet. Drizzle with a little olive oil. Bake for 12-15 minutes, or until the salmon is cooked through and easily flakes with a fork.

3. While the salmon is baking, prepare the mango salsa. In a bowl, combine the diced

mango, red onion, cilantro, lime juice, and jalapeño (if using). Mix well and season with salt to taste. Set aside.

4. Cook the quinoa according to package instructions. Fluff with a fork when done.

5. To serve, divide the cooked quinoa among plates. Top each portion with a baked salmon fillet and a generous spoonful of the mango salsa. Enjoy immediately.

Nutritional Information (per serving):

- Calories: 380
- Fat: 16g
- Saturated Fat: 3g
- Carbohydrates: 28g
- Fiber: 4g
- Protein: 32g

Dietary Recommendations

Salmon is an excellent protein choice for those with myasthenia gravis. It is soft, easy to chew, and packed with healthy omega-3 fatty acids which may help reduce inflammation. Baking the salmon ensures a moist and tender texture. The mango salsa adds a bright, fresh flavor and a boost of nutrients. Mango is rich in vitamins A and C, while cilantro and lime juice provide additional antioxidants. The salsa can be made milder by omitting the jalapeño if spice is a concern.

Quinoa is a nutritious gluten-free grain that is high in protein and fiber. Its soft texture makes it easy to eat for those with swallowing difficulties. Cook the quinoa in broth instead of water for added flavor if desired. This well-rounded meal offers a balance of protein, healthy fats, and complex carbohydrates to provide sustained energy throughout the day. Feel free to adjust portions based on your individual needs and appetite.

Greek Quinoa Salad with Grilled Chicken

Ingredients:

- 1 cup quinoa, rinsed and drained
- 2 cups water
- 2 boneless, skinless chicken breasts
- 1 pint cherry tomatoes, halved
- 1 cucumber, diced
- 1/2 red onion, finely chopped
- 1/2 cup crumbled feta cheese
- 1/2 cup pitted Kalamata olives, halved
- 1/4 cup Greek dressing

Step-by-Step Preparation Instructions:

1. In a medium saucepan, combine the quinoa and water. Bring to a boil, then reduce heat to low, cover, and simmer for 15 minutes or until the water is absorbed. Fluff the quinoa with a fork and set aside to cool.

2. Preheat your grill or grill pan to medium-high heat. Season the chicken breasts with salt and pepper. Grill the chicken for 6-8 minutes per side or until cooked through. Let the chicken rest for 5 minutes before slicing.

3. In a large bowl, combine the cooled quinoa, sliced chicken, cherry tomatoes, cucumber, red onion, feta cheese, and Kalamata olives.

4. Drizzle the Greek dressing over the salad and toss gently to combine. For added flavor, you can add freshly chopped herbs like parsley or oregano.

5. Serve the salad immediately, or refrigerate for up to 2 hours before serving.

Nutritional Information (per serving):

- Calories: 350
- Total Fat: 12g
- Saturated Fat: 3g
- Cholesterol: 65mg
- Sodium: 520mg
- Total Carbohydrates: 35g
- Dietary Fiber: 5g
- Protein: 28g

Dietary Recommendation

This Greek Quinoa Salad with Grilled Chicken is a nutritious and flavorful meal that aligns well with the dietary guidelines for individuals with myasthenia gravis. Quinoa provides complex carbohydrates and fiber, while the grilled chicken offers lean protein. The vegetables contribute essential vitamins and minerals.

To make this recipe even more MG-friendly, consider using a low-fat Greek dressing to reduce the overall fat content. You can also chop the vegetables and chicken into smaller pieces to make chewing and swallowing easier if needed. Feel free to adjust the ingredients based on your personal preferences and dietary requirements.

Roasted Vegetable and Egg Breakfast Sandwiches

Ingredients:

- 4 whole-grain bread slices
- 2 bell peppers, sliced
- 1 zucchini, sliced
- 4 eggs
- 1 avocado, mashed
- Salt and pepper to taste

Step-by-Step Preparation Instructions:

1. Preheat your oven to 425°F (220°C). Line a baking sheet with parchment paper.

2. Arrange the sliced bell peppers and zucchini on the prepared baking sheet. Drizzle with olive oil and season with salt and pepper. Roast the vegetables for 20-25 minutes, or until tender and lightly caramelized.

3. While the vegetables are roasting, prepare the

eggs. Heat a non-stick skillet over medium heat. Crack the eggs into the skillet and cook until the whites are set and the yolks are cooked to your desired doneness. Season with salt and pepper.

4. Toast the whole-grain bread slices until golden brown.

5. To assemble the sandwiches, spread the mashed avocado evenly on two bread slices. Top with the roasted vegetables and cooked eggs. Place the remaining bread slices on top to complete the sandwiches.

6. Serve the sandwiches immediately while the vegetables and eggs are still warm. For added flavor, you can sprinkle fresh herbs like basil or cilantro on top.

Nutritional Information (per serving):

- Calories: 400
- Total Fat: 20g
- Saturated Fat: 4g
- Cholesterol: 370mg
- Sodium: 420mg
- Total Carbohydrates: 38g
- Dietary Fiber: 9g
- Protein: 19g

Dietary Recommendation

These Roasted Vegetable and Egg Breakfast Sandwiches provide a balanced meal to start your day. The whole-grain bread offers complex carbohydrates and fiber, while the eggs and avocado contribute protein and healthy fats. The roasted vegetables add valuable nutrients and antioxidants. To make this recipe more suitable for individuals with swallowing difficulties, you can mash the roasted vegetables and eggs together before spreading them on the bread. This creates a softer, more manageable texture. You can also cut the sandwiches into smaller pieces for easier consumption.

Vegetable and Tofu Stir-Fry with Brown Rice Noodles and Peanut Sauce

Ingredients:

- 14 oz extra-firm tofu, drained and cubed
- 4 cups mixed vegetables (such as broccoli, bell peppers, carrots, and snap peas)
- 8 oz brown rice noodles
- 2 cloves garlic, minced
- 1 tbsp fresh ginger, grated
- 1/4 cup low-sodium soy sauce
- 1/4 cup creamy peanut butter
- 2 tbsp lime juice
- 2 tbsp vegetable oil
- Salt and pepper to taste
- Optional garnish: chopped peanuts, fresh cilantro

Preparation:

1. Press the tofu between two plates lined with paper towels to remove excess moisture. Cut into 1-inch cubes and set aside.

2. Cook the brown rice noodles according to package instructions. Drain and rinse with cold water.

3. In a small bowl, whisk together the soy sauce, peanut butter, lime juice, garlic, and ginger until smooth. Set the peanut sauce aside.

4. Heat the vegetable oil in a large wok or skillet over medium-high heat. Add the tofu cubes and stir-fry for 5 minutes until lightly golden. Season with salt and pepper.

5. Add the mixed vegetables to the pan and stir-fry for an additional 5-7 minutes until crisp-tender.

6. Pour the peanut sauce over the tofu and vegetables, stirring to coat evenly. Cook for 2-3 minutes until heated through.

7. Divide the cooked brown rice noodles among serving bowls. Top with the vegetable and tofu stir-fry.

8. Garnish with chopped peanuts and fresh cilantro if desired. Serve hot and enjoy the delightful blend of flavors and textures in this nutritious and satisfying dish.

Nutritional Information (per serving): Calories: 450 Total Fat: 22g Saturated Fat: 3g Cholesterol: 0mg Sodium: 620mg Total Carbohydrate: 48g Dietary Fiber: 8g Sugars: 6g Protein: 22g

Dietary Recommendation

This vegetable and tofu stir-fry with brown rice noodles

and peanut sauce is a wholesome and delicious option for those following a vegetarian or vegan diet. The dish is packed with fiber, plant-based protein, and essential vitamins and minerals from the colorful mix of vegetables.

The tofu provides a lean protein source that is gentle on the digestive system, making it suitable for individuals with Myasthenia Gravis who may experience difficulty chewing or swallowing. The brown rice noodles offer a gluten-free alternative to traditional wheat-based noodles, catering to those with gluten sensitivities. To enhance the flavors and make the dish even more appealing, consider adding a splash of rice vinegar or a sprinkle of red pepper flakes to the peanut sauce for a tangy kick or a hint of heat. Feel free to customize the vegetable mix based on your preferences or seasonal availability, ensuring a vibrant and nutrient-rich meal every time.

Grilled Salmon and Asparagus Salad with Lemon Vinaigrette and Quinoa

Ingredients:

- 4 (6 oz) salmon fillets
- 1 bunch asparagus, trimmed
- 4 cups mixed greens
- 1 cup cherry tomatoes, halved
- 1 cup cooked quinoa
- 2 tbsp olive oil
- Salt and pepper to taste

Lemon Vinaigrette:

- 1/4 cup olive oil
- 2 tbsp fresh lemon juice
- 1 tsp Dijon mustard
- 1 clove garlic, minced
- Salt and pepper to taste

Preparation:

1. Preheat the grill to medium-high heat. Brush the salmon fillets and asparagus with olive oil and season with salt and pepper.

2. Grill the salmon for 4-5 minutes per side, or until it flakes easily with a fork. Simultaneously, grill the asparagus for 5-7 minutes, turning occasionally, until tender and lightly charred. Remove from the grill and set aside.

3. In a small bowl, whisk together the olive oil, lemon juice, Dijon mustard, minced garlic, salt, and pepper to make the lemon vinaigrette. Adjust the seasoning to taste.

4. In a large bowl, combine the mixed greens,

cherry tomatoes, and cooked quinoa. Toss gently to mix.

5. Divide the salad mixture among serving plates. Top each salad with a grilled salmon fillet and a portion of the grilled asparagus.

6. Drizzle the lemon vinaigrette over the salads, ensuring an even distribution of the tangy and zesty flavors.

7. Serve the grilled salmon and asparagus salad immediately, allowing the warmth of the salmon and asparagus to gently wilt the mixed greens. Savor the harmonious combination of flavors and textures in every bite.

Nutritional Information (per serving): Calories: 480 Total Fat: 29g Saturated Fat: 4g Cholesterol: 80mg Sodium: 320mg Total Carbohydrate: 21g Dietary Fiber: 5g Sugars: 4g Protein: 37g

Dietary Recommendation

This grilled salmon and asparagus salad with lemon vinaigrette and quinoa is an ideal choice for individuals seeking a nutritious and flavorful meal that supports their overall well-being, especially those managing Myasthenia Gravis. Salmon is an excellent source of omega-3 fatty acids, which have anti-inflammatory properties and may help alleviate muscle weakness associated with the condition.

Asparagus is a nutrient-dense vegetable that provides a

good amount of fiber, vitamins, and minerals, promoting digestive health and overall nourishment. The mixed greens and cherry tomatoes add a refreshing lightness to the dish, while the quinoa contributes a protein-rich and gluten-free carbohydrate source. To elevate the flavors and make the dish even more enticing, consider adding fresh herbs like dill or basil to the lemon vinaigrette for an extra layer of freshness. If desired, you can also sprinkle some toasted almonds or pumpkin seeds over the salad for a delightful crunch and an additional boost of healthy fats and nutrients.

Quinoa and Black Bean Stuffed Bell Peppers with Avocado Salsa

Ingredients:

- 4 large bell peppers (any color)
- 1 cup uncooked quinoa, rinsed
- 2 cups vegetable broth or water
- 1 can (15 oz) black beans, drained and rinsed
- 1 can (14.5 oz) diced tomatoes, drained
- 1/2 cup diced onion
- 3 cloves garlic, minced
- 1 tsp ground cumin
- Salt and pepper to taste
- Avocado Salsa (see recipe below)

Preparation Instructions:

1. Preheat the oven to 375°F (190°C).

2. Cut the tops off the bell peppers and remove the seeds and membranes. Place the peppers cut-side up in a baking dish and set aside.

3. In a medium saucepan, combine the quinoa and vegetable broth (or water). Bring to a boil over high heat. Reduce heat to low, cover, and simmer until quinoa is tender and liquid is absorbed, about 15-20 minutes.

4. In a large bowl, combine the cooked quinoa, black beans, diced tomatoes, onion, garlic, cumin, salt and pepper. Mix until well combined.

5. Spoon the quinoa mixture into the bell peppers, mounding it slightly. Cover the baking dish with foil.

6. Bake for 30 minutes. Remove the foil and bake for an additional 15-20 minutes, until the peppers are tender and lightly browned on top.

7. Serve the stuffed peppers hot, topped with a generous spoonful of Avocado Salsa.

Avocado Salsa:

- 2 ripe avocados, diced
- 1/2 cup diced red onion
- 1 small jalapeño pepper, seeded and minced
- 1/4 cup chopped fresh cilantro
- Juice of 1 lime

- Salt to taste

In a medium bowl, gently mix together all ingredients for the salsa. Cover and refrigerate until ready to serve.

Nutritional Information (per stuffed pepper):

- Calories: 320
- Total Fat: 11g
- Saturated Fat: 1.5g
- Cholesterol: 0mg
- Sodium: 400mg
- Total Carbohydrates: 48g
- Dietary Fiber: 13g
- Total Sugars: 5g
- Protein: 12g

Dietary Recommendations

This hearty and flavorful dish is rich in protein, fiber, and essential nutrients, making it an excellent choice for those following a myasthenia gravis diet. Quinoa provides high-quality plant-based protein, while black beans offer additional protein and fiber. The bell peppers, tomatoes, and avocado salsa contribute vitamin C, potassium, and healthy fats.

To make this dish easier to eat for those with swallowing difficulties, the bell peppers can be chopped into smaller pieces before stuffing. The quinoa and bean filling can also be mashed slightly for a softer texture. For a flavor boost, consider adding a sprinkle of smoked paprika or a dash of hot sauce to the filling mixture before baking.

Enjoy this colorful and satisfying meal as a nourishing lunch or dinner option.

Baked Chicken with Roasted Brussels Sprouts, Sweet Potatoes, and Balsamic Glaze

Ingredients:

- 4 boneless, skinless chicken breasts
- 1 lb Brussels sprouts, trimmed and halved
- 2 medium sweet potatoes, peeled and cut into 1-inch cubes
- 2 tbsp olive oil, divided
- 4 cloves garlic, minced
- Salt and pepper to taste
- 1/4 cup balsamic vinegar
- 2 tbsp honey

Preparation Instructions:

1. Preheat the oven to 400°F (200°C).

2. In a large bowl, toss the Brussels sprouts and sweet potatoes with 1 tablespoon of olive oil, half of the minced garlic, salt, and pepper. Spread the vegetables in a single layer on a large baking sheet.

3. Season the chicken breasts with salt and pepper. Heat the remaining tablespoon of olive oil in a large oven-safe skillet over medium-high heat. Add the chicken and cook until golden brown, about 3-4 minutes per side.

4. Transfer the skillet with the chicken to the oven, and place the baking sheet with the

vegetables on a separate rack. Bake for 20-25 minutes, until the chicken is cooked through (internal temperature reaches 165°F/74°C) and the vegetables are tender and caramelized.

5. While the chicken and vegetables are baking, prepare the balsamic glaze: In a small saucepan, combine the balsamic vinegar, honey, and remaining minced garlic. Bring to a boil over medium-high heat, then reduce heat to low and simmer until the glaze has thickened and reduced by half, about 5-7 minutes.

6. Remove the chicken and vegetables from the oven. Let the chicken rest for 5 minutes before slicing.

7. Divide the sliced chicken and roasted vegetables among 4 plates. Drizzle the balsamic glaze over the chicken and vegetables, and serve hot.

Nutritional Information (per serving):

- Calories: 380
- Total Fat: 11g
- Saturated Fat: 2g
- Cholesterol: 85mg
- Sodium: 300mg
- Total Carbohydrates: 38g
- Dietary Fiber: 7g
- Total Sugars: 17g
- Protein: 34g

Dietary Recommendations

This well-rounded meal features lean protein from the chicken, fiber and antioxidants from the Brussels sprouts and sweet potatoes, and a flavorful balsamic glaze to tie it all together. The combination of ingredients provides a variety of essential nutrients, including vitamins A and C, potassium, and iron.

To ensure that this dish is suitable for those with myasthenia gravis, the chicken can be cut into smaller, bite-sized pieces before cooking to make it easier to chew and swallow. The Brussels sprouts and sweet potatoes should be cooked until very tender, and can be mashed slightly with a fork if needed. The balsamic glaze adds a delightful sweet-tart flavor to the dish, but can be omitted or served on the side if desired. For an extra boost of nutrition and flavor, consider adding a sprinkle of chopped fresh herbs like rosemary or thyme to the vegetables before roasting. This comforting and nourishing meal is perfect for a cozy dinner at home, and any leftovers can be easily reheated for a quick and satisfying lunch the next day.

Vegetable and Lentil Soup with Pesto and Whole-Grain Crackers

Ingredients:

- 1 cup dried green or brown lentils, rinsed

- 1 can (14.5 oz) diced tomatoes, undrained
- 2 medium carrots, diced
- 2 celery stalks, diced
- 1 medium onion, chopped
- 3 garlic cloves, minced
- 6 cups low-sodium vegetable broth
- 2 tablespoons pesto sauce
- Salt and black pepper to taste
- Whole-grain crackers for serving

Preparation Instructions:

1. In a large pot, combine the lentils, diced tomatoes with their juice, carrots, celery, onion, garlic, and vegetable broth. Bring to a boil over high heat.

2. Reduce the heat to low, cover the pot, and simmer for about 30-35 minutes or until the lentils and vegetables are tender.

3. Remove from heat and stir in the pesto sauce. Season with salt and pepper to taste.

4. Serve hot with whole-grain crackers on the side.

Flavor Enhancer: For added depth of flavor, consider stirring in 1 tablespoon of balsamic vinegar or 1 teaspoon of smoked paprika along with the pesto sauce.

Nutritional Information (per serving, based on 6 servings):

- Calories: 210
- Total Fat: 4g

- Saturated Fat: 1g
- Cholesterol: 0mg
- Sodium: 280mg
- Total Carbohydrates: 34g
- Dietary Fiber: 11g
- Sugars: 5g
- Protein: 12g

Dietary Recommendations

This hearty vegetable and lentil soup is a nutritious choice for those with Myasthenia Gravis. Lentils provide a good source of plant-based protein, fiber, and essential nutrients like iron and folate. The vegetables offer added fiber, vitamins, and minerals. The pesto sauce adds a flavorful twist while keeping the soup easy to swallow. Serve with soft, whole-grain crackers for a satisfying meal that's gentle on the digestive system.

Mediterranean Chickpea Salad with Grilled Shrimp and Feta

Ingredients:

- 1 can (15 oz) chickpeas, rinsed and drained
- 1 pint cherry tomatoes, halved
- 1 English cucumber, diced

- 1/2 red onion, thinly sliced
- 1/2 cup crumbled feta cheese
- 1/4 cup chopped fresh parsley
- 2 tablespoons lemon juice
- 2 tablespoons extra-virgin olive oil
- Salt and black pepper to taste
- 1 pound medium shrimp, peeled and deveined
- 1 tablespoon olive oil
- 1 teaspoon dried oregano

Preparation Instructions:

1. In a large bowl, combine the chickpeas, cherry tomatoes, cucumber, red onion, feta cheese, and parsley.

2. In a small bowl, whisk together the lemon juice and extra-virgin olive oil. Season with salt and pepper to taste.

3. Pour the dressing over the salad and toss gently to combine. Set aside.

4. Preheat a grill or grill pan over medium-high heat.

5. In a bowl, toss the shrimp with olive oil, oregano, salt, and pepper.

6. Grill the shrimp for 2-3 minutes per side or until pink and cooked through.

7. Serve the grilled shrimp on top of the Mediterranean chickpea salad.

Nutritional Information (per serving, based on 4 servings):

- Calories: 370
- Total Fat: 16g
- Saturated Fat: 4g
- Cholesterol: 180mg
- Sodium: 620mg
- Total Carbohydrates: 28g
- Dietary Fiber: 8g
- Sugars: 6g
- Protein: 30g

Dietary Recommendations

This Mediterranean-inspired chickpea salad with grilled shrimp is a protein-rich and flavorful dish suitable for those with Myasthenia Gravis. Chickpeas and shrimp provide lean protein, while the vegetables offer fiber, vitamins, and minerals. The feta cheese adds a creamy, tangy element that complements the other ingredients. The dressing is light and refreshing, making this salad easy to eat and digest. Grilling the shrimp keeps the dish tender and flavorful without the need for heavy sauces or seasonings.

Quinoa and Roasted Vegetable Grain Bowls with Avocado

Ingredients:

- 1 cup quinoa, rinsed
- 2 cups water
- 1 head broccoli, cut into florets
- 1 head cauliflower, cut into florets

- 2 bell peppers, sliced
- 4 cloves garlic, minced
- 2 tablespoons olive oil
- Juice of 1 lemon
- 1/2 cup crumbled feta cheese
- 1 avocado, sliced

Preparation Instructions:

1. Preheat your oven to 425°F (220°C). Line a baking sheet with parchment paper.

2. In a medium pot, bring the quinoa and water to a boil. Reduce the heat to low, cover, and simmer for 15 minutes or until the water is absorbed and the quinoa is fluffy.

3. Meanwhile, in a large bowl, toss the broccoli, cauliflower, bell peppers, and garlic with the olive oil. Spread the vegetables on the prepared baking sheet and roast for 20-25 minutes, stirring halfway through, until tender and lightly charred.

4. Once the quinoa is cooked, fluff it with a fork and transfer to a large serving bowl. Add the roasted vegetables, lemon juice, and feta cheese. Gently toss to combine.

5. Divide the quinoa and vegetable mixture among four bowls. Top each bowl with sliced avocado. For an extra burst of flavor, drizzle with additional olive oil and sprinkle with salt and pepper to taste.

Nutritional Information (per serving):

- Calories: 450
- Total Fat: 22g
- Saturated Fat: 5g
- Cholesterol: 17mg
- Sodium: 280mg
- Total Carbohydrates: 52g
- Dietary Fiber: 12g
- Sugars: 6g
- Protein: 15g

Dietary Recommendations

This quinoa and roasted vegetable grain bowl is a nutritious and delicious option for those with Myasthenia Gravis. Quinoa provides complex carbohydrates and protein, while the roasted vegetables offer a variety of vitamins, minerals, and fiber. The healthy fats from the olive oil and avocado promote satiety and support overall health. The soft texture of the quinoa and roasted vegetables makes this dish easy to chew and swallow, which is important for those experiencing muscle weakness. The lemon juice and feta cheese add a bright, tangy flavor that enhances the natural taste of the vegetables without the need for excess salt or heavy sauces.

Baked Cod with Tomato and Olive Tapenade and Roasted Potatoes

Ingredients:

- 4 cod fillets (6 oz each)

- 1 can (14.5 oz) diced tomatoes, drained
- 1/2 cup pitted Kalamata olives, chopped
- 2 cloves garlic, minced
- 2 tablespoons olive oil, divided
- 1/4 cup fresh basil, chopped
- 2 tablespoons capers, drained
- 1 pound baby potatoes, halved
- Salt and pepper to taste

Preparation Instructions:

1. Preheat your oven to 400°F (200°C). Line a baking sheet with parchment paper.

2. In a bowl, combine the drained diced tomatoes, chopped olives, minced garlic, 1 tablespoon of olive oil, chopped basil, and capers. Mix well to create the tapenade.

3. Place the halved baby potatoes on the prepared baking sheet. Drizzle with the remaining 1 tablespoon of olive oil and season with salt and pepper. Toss to coat evenly. Roast the potatoes for 25-30 minutes, or until tender and golden brown, stirring halfway through.

4. While the potatoes are roasting, season the cod fillets with salt and pepper on both sides. Place them in a baking dish and top each fillet with a generous spoonful of the tomato and olive tapenade.

5. Bake the cod fillets for 12-15 minutes, or until the fish is cooked through and flakes easily with a fork. The internal temperature should

reach 145°F (63°C).

6. Serve the baked cod fillets with the roasted potatoes on the side. Garnish with additional fresh basil if desired.

Nutritional Information (per serving):

- Calories: 380
- Total Fat: 15g
- Saturated Fat: 2g
- Cholesterol: 65mg
- Sodium: 520mg
- Total Carbohydrates: 28g
- Dietary Fiber: 4g
- Sugars: 3g
- Protein: 32g

Dietary Recommendations

This baked cod recipe is an excellent choice for those with Myasthenia Gravis due to its soft texture and nutrient-dense ingredients. Cod is a lean protein source that is easy to chew and swallow, while the tomato and olive tapenade provides a flavorful topping rich in antioxidants and healthy fats.

The roasted potatoes offer a comforting and nutritious side dish that is soft and easy to eat. The olive oil used in the recipe provides monounsaturated fats, which are beneficial for heart health and can help reduce inflammation. To ensure a moist and tender result, be cautious not to overcook the cod fillets. The dish can be adapted to your taste preferences by adjusting the amount of garlic, olives, or capers in the tapenade. For a pop of color and added nutrients, consider serving the cod and potatoes with a side of steamed green vegetables like spinach or green beans.

Spinach and Feta Stuffed Chicken Breasts with Roasted Vegetables

Ingredients:

- 4 boneless, skinless chicken breasts
- 2 cups fresh spinach, chopped
- 1/2 cup crumbled feta cheese
- 1/2 onion, finely diced
- 2 cloves garlic, minced
- 2 tbsp olive oil, divided
- 2 cups mixed vegetables (such as zucchini, bell peppers, and carrots), chopped
- Salt and pepper to taste

Preparation:

1. Preheat your oven to 400°F (200°C).

2. In a medium bowl, mix together the chopped spinach, feta cheese, diced onion, minced garlic, 1 tablespoon of olive oil, and a pinch of salt and pepper until well combined. This filling is bursting with Mediterranean flavors that will elevate your chicken to new heights.

3. Carefully butterfly each chicken breast, making a pocket to hold the filling. Spoon a quarter of the spinach and feta mixture into each chicken breast pocket. Secure with toothpicks if needed. Season the outside of the chicken with salt and pepper.

4. In a large oven-safe skillet or baking dish, toss the chopped mixed vegetables with the remaining 1 tablespoon of olive oil and a sprinkle of salt and pepper. Nestle the stuffed chicken breasts among the vegetables.

5. Roast in the preheated oven for 25-30 minutes, until the chicken is cooked through (internal temperature reaches 165°F/74°C) and the vegetables are tender and lightly caramelized. The aroma wafting from your oven will have your mouth watering in anticipation.

6. Remove from the oven and let the chicken rest for 5 minutes before serving. Serve the stuffed chicken breasts hot, surrounded by the flavorful roasted vegetables. Each bite is a delightful combination of juicy chicken, creamy feta, vibrant spinach, and sweet roasted veggies.

Nutritional Information (per serving): Calories: 350 Protein: 38g Carbohydrates: 8g Fat: 18g Fiber: 3g

Grilled Veggie and Hummus Wraps with Quinoa

Ingredients:

- 4 whole-wheat tortillas
- 1 cup hummus
- 1 zucchini, sliced lengthwise
- 1 red bell pepper, cut into strips
- 1 yellow bell pepper, cut into strips
- 1 onion, sliced into rings
- 2 cups mixed greens
- 1 cup cooked quinoa
- 2 tbsp olive oil
- Salt and pepper to taste

Preparation:

1. Preheat your grill or grill pan to medium-high heat.

2. Brush the sliced zucchini, bell peppers, and onion with olive oil and season with salt and pepper. Grill the vegetables for 5-7 minutes per side, until they are tender and have nice grill marks. The smoky flavor imparted by the grill takes these simple veggies to a whole new level of deliciousness.

3. Warm the tortillas on the grill for about 30 seconds per side, just until they're pliable and have a few light grill marks.

4. To assemble the wraps, spread about 1/4 cup of hummus down the center of each warm tortilla. Add a quarter of the grilled vegetables, 1/2 cup of mixed greens, and 1/4 cup of cooked quinoa to each wrap.

The combination of creamy hummus, smoky grilled veggies, fresh greens, and nutty quinoa creates a symphony of flavors and textures.

5. Fold the sides of the tortilla over the filling, then roll up tightly to form a wrap. Slice in half diagonally and serve immediately. These wraps are a feast for the eyes as well as the palate, with their vibrant colors and enticing aroma.

Nutritional Information (per wrap): Calories: 400 Protein: 14g

Carbohydrates: 56g Fat: 15g Fiber: 11g

Sweet Potato and Black Bean Burrito Bowls with Brown Rice

Dive into a vibrant medley of flavors and textures with these nourishing Sweet Potato and Black Bean Burrito Bowls. Roasted sweet potatoes, protein-packed black beans, and wholesome brown rice come together in a symphony of tastes, while fresh avocado, zesty salsa, tangy lime juice, and fragrant cilantro elevate each bite. This dish not only tantalizes your taste buds but also provides a balanced meal that supports your overall well-being and energy levels.

Ingredients list:

- 2 medium sweet potatoes, peeled and diced into 1-inch cubes
- 1 tablespoon olive oil
- Salt and pepper to taste
- 1 cup cooked black beans, rinsed and drained
- 1 cup cooked brown rice
- 1 ripe avocado, diced
- 1/2 cup salsa of your choice
- Juice of 1 lime
- Fresh cilantro, chopped (optional)

Step-by-step preparation instructions:

1. Preheat your oven to 400°F (200°C).

2. In a large bowl, toss the diced sweet potatoes with olive oil, salt, and pepper until evenly coated.

3. Spread the seasoned sweet potatoes on a baking sheet lined with parchment paper and roast for 25-30 minutes, or until tender and lightly caramelized. Stir halfway through for even cooking.

4. While the sweet potatoes are roasting, prepare the black beans and brown rice according to package instructions if not already cooked.

5. Once the sweet potatoes are done, assemble your burrito bowls by dividing the brown rice evenly among 2-3 bowls.

6. Top each bowl with roasted sweet potatoes, black beans, diced avocado, and a generous spoonful of salsa.

7. Drizzle fresh lime juice over each bowl for a zesty kick.

8. Garnish with chopped cilantro for added freshness and flavor, if desired.

9. Serve your Sweet Potato and Black Bean Burrito Bowls immediately and enjoy the harmonious blend of flavors and textures.

Flavor Enhancer Tip: For an extra depth of flavor, consider adding a sprinkle of cumin, smoked paprika, or chili powder to the sweet potatoes before roasting.

Recipe Nutritional Information (per serving, based on 2 servings):

- Calories: 520
- Protein: 16g
- Total Fat: 20g
- Saturated Fat: 3g
- Carbohydrates: 75g
- Fiber: 18g
- Sugar: 8g
- Sodium: 480mg

Dietary Recommendation

This Sweet Potato and Black Bean Burrito Bowl is a nutritious and satisfying meal that aligns with the dietary guidelines for individuals with Myasthenia Gravis. The dish incorporates a variety of nourishing ingredients, including fiber-rich sweet potatoes, protein-packed black beans, and wholesome brown rice. The avocado provides healthy fats, while the salsa and lime juice add vibrant flavors without relying on excessive salt or sugar. The soft, easy-to-chew textures of the roasted sweet potatoes, black beans, and avocado make this dish suitable for those who may experience difficulty swallowing. The moisture from the salsa and lime juice further enhances the ease of consumption.

CONCLUSION

In conclusion, it takes resiliency, persistence, and a thorough awareness of the disease itself to live with Myasthenia Gravis. It is a complicated and varied journey. Through this thorough guide, we have walked you through the complexities of this neuromuscular condition, revealing its mysterious nature and giving you the information and resources you need to take back control of your health.

From the historical origins of Myasthenia Gravis to its diverse manifestations, including ocular, generalized, and seronegative forms, this book has served as a beacon of enlightenment, shedding light on the complexities that often shroud this invisible illness. We have delved into the intricate mechanisms that underlie the diagnosis process, decoding the crucial role of acetylcholine receptor antibodies and the nuances of distinguishing between various subtypes.

Recognizing the urgency of managing exacerbations and crises, we have armed you with strategies to navigate these challenging moments, empowering you to confront them with confidence and preparedness.

Furthermore, we have explored the vast array of treatment options available, from mainstream medications to unconventional therapies, emphasizing the importance of individualized care and vigilant medication management. The transformative potential of Thymectomy has been highlighted, providing you with a comprehensive understanding of its role in managing Myasthenia Gravis and its associated thymomas. This knowledge serves as a powerful tool in making informed decisions about your healthcare journey.

Extending beyond the realm of medical interventions, this guide has become a sanctuary of practical wisdom, offering advice on nutrition, physical therapy, and self-care strategies tailored to elevate your quality of life and alleviate the invisible symptoms of this condition. We have navigated the treacherous terrain of medications to avoid, ensuring your well-being remains the highest priority. This book has shed light on the fascinating field of continuing research, upcoming novel treatments, and the fascinating world of clinical trials as we look to the future. It has given us a view into the seemingly endless possibilities for improvements in the treatment of Myasthenia Gravis. As a result, ***Myasthenia Gravis: A Complete Guide to Understanding, Managing, and Driving Myasthenia Gravis into Remission with Delicious Anti-Inflammatory Recipes and Diet Plans*** has been a thorough companion that has given you the information, techniques, and steadfast support you need to deal with the challenges of this long-term condition. Equipped with this priceless tool, you can set out on a path of self-actualization, meeting the obstacles posed by Myasthenia Gravis with fortitude, optimism, and a resolute dedication to leading a satisfying life.